D1136749

EPIDEMIOLOGY OF MENTAL DISORDERS
AND PSYCHOSOCIAL PROBLEMS

Schizophrenia

Richard Warner
Medical Director
Mental Health Center of Boulder County and
Associate Professor
University of Colorado
Boulder, CO, USA

Giovanni de Girolamo
Division of Mental Health
World Health Organization
Geneva, Switzerland

World Health Organization
Geneva
1995

WHO Library Cataloguing in Publication Data
Warner, Richard.
  Schizophrenia / Richard Warner, Giovanni de Girolamo.
  (Epidemiology of mental disorders and psychosocial problems)
  1.Schizophrenia I.De Girolamo, Giovanni II.Series

  ISBN 92 4 156171 8   (NLM Classification: WM 203)

The World Health Organization welcomes requests for permission to reproduce or translate its publications, in part or in full. Applications and enquiries should be addressed to the Office of Publications, World Health Organization, Geneva, Switzerland, which will be glad to provide the latest information on any changes made to the text, plans for new editions, and reprints and translations already available.

© World Health Organization 1995

The designations employed and the presentation of the material in this publication do not imply the expression of any opinion whatsoever on the part of the Secretariat of the World Health Organization concerning the legal status of any country, territory, city or area or of its authorities, or concerning the delimitation of its frontiers or boundaries.

The mention of specific companies or of certain manufacturers' products does not imply that they are endorsed or recommended by the World Health Organization in preference to others of a similar nature that are not mentioned. Errors and omissions excepted, the names of proprietary products are distinguished by initial capital letters.

The authors alone are responsible for the views expressed in this publication.

TYPESET IN INDIA
PRINTED IN ENGLAND
93/9891-Macmillan/Clays-7500

Contents

Preface

Psychiatric illness is common and can have serious consequences. It has been estimated that as many as 500 million people may be suffering from some kind of mental disorder or impairment (WHO, 1992a). In many countries 40% of disabled people owe their disability to mental disorders. Epidemiological predictions concerning mental illness show that there is every probability that the magnitude of mental health problems will increase in the future, as a result of various factors, including the increasing life expectancy of those with a mental disorder or disability and the growing number of people reaching the ages in which the risk of mental disorder is high.

The magnitude of mental health problems far exceeds that of the resources available for their resolution. In most parts of the world services which could help people who suffer from mental disorders are insufficient in both quality and quantity. This is often true even in the most highly developed countries. The general public and most of the professional medical community—often including psychiatrists—are insufficiently aware of the extent and nature of mental disorders and of the burden which these disorders represent for the individuals who suffer from them, their families and their communities. Traditional health statistical services in most countries are unable to provide accurate information about the extent of mental health problems in their populations. Most statistics routinely collected by health statistical services are based on mortality, which may lead to a distorted picture of the health status of a population since diseases of long duration that do not necessarily end in death—including many mental and neurological conditions—do not show up in such statistics. Lack of awareness of the magnitude and nature of mental health problems and of the availability of effective means of preventing or treating them is the cause of the low priority given to mental health programmes in most countries.

If health priorities are to be chosen properly, it is essential for accurate information to be available on the incidence and prevalence of mental and neurological disorders in the community and in general health facilities, their variation across countries and cultures and over time, their sociodemographic characteristics and the risk factors associated with their occurrence.

Unfortunately, reliable and comparable epidemiological data on mental and neurological disorders are scarce. Two of the reasons for the paucity of such data are particularly important: (1) the inadequacy of the training received by general health care personnel (and the absence of biological markers of mental illness) leads to a low recognition rate of mental health problems in their patients; and (2) the absence until recently of a "common language"—comprising a nomenclature, an agreed diagnostic system, and standardized instruments for the assessment of these disorders—means that the data that have been collected are not truly comparable.

Ideally, a series of cross-cultural surveys should be carried out for well-defined conditions or groups of conditions in order to advance our knowledge of the epidemiology of mental health problems. Over the past 20 years considerable progress has been made in developing the methodology for carrying out such work. WHO has played an important role in this field: with the publication of diagnostic guidelines accompanying Chapter V of ICD-10 (WHO, 1992b), a widely tested and accepted diagnostic system has become available; WHO has also contributed to the development of instruments for the standardized assessment of psychopathology, including the Composite International Diagnostic Interview (CIDI) (Robins et al., 1988), the Schedules for Clinical Assessment in Neuropsychiatry (SCAN) (Wing et al., 1990), and the International Personality Disorder Examination (IPDE) (Loranger et al., 1991), and developed a network of centres in which training in their use can be obtained. In addition, WHO has carried out cross-cultural clinical and epidemiological research which has demonstrated that such work is feasible, and established research teams and centres in which further related work can be carried out.

Some countries have conducted major epidemiological studies in recent years (e.g. Brazil, China, USA), but data on the epidemiology of mental disorders are still scarce and difficult to obtain. For these reasons, WHO decided to produce a series of monographs, each of which discusses epidemiological data on a specific disorder (or group of related disorders). Special attention is given to epidemiological data gathered in developing countries, which are often neglected in epidemiological reviews published in scientific journals. As shown in several major WHO epidemiological studies (e.g. the International Pilot Study of Schizophrenia (WHO, 1979); the study on depression in different cultures (Sartorius et al., 1983); the study on the determinants of the outcome of severe mental disorders (Jablensky et al., 1992); the study on pathways to psychiatric care (Gater et al., 1991); and the study on ill-defined psychological disorders in general medical settings (Sartorius et al., 1990)), the comparison of epidemiological data obtained in developing countries, or in countries that do not have a long tradition of epidemiological research, with those gathered in developed countries, or in countries with a stronger tradition of such research, can provide valuable insights into the very nature of the disorders—their causes, form, course and outcome.

All these monographs are similar in format: they review issues related to diagnosis and classification, with special reference to ICD-10, as well as the standardized instruments available and used for the assessment of mental disorders. Incidence and prevalence studies carried out in the general population, in primary care settings, and in psychiatric settings, as well as in other institutions such as nursing homes, prisons, etc., are also reviewed. The main risk factors for the disorder, or group of disorders, are then discussed, and data on time trends in the prevalence and incidence of the disorder given where available. Each monograph ends with conclusions and recommendations for future studies.

It is hoped that these monographs will help research and health institutions, health planners, clinicians, and those concerned with informing the general public to understand better the magnitude of the problems they have to face, to develop effective preventive strategies and to build appropriate and humane care-delivery systems.

W. Gulbinat
Division of Mental Health
World Health Organization

References

Gater R et al. (1991) The pathway study. *Psychological medicine*, 21: 761–774.

Jablensky A et al. (1992) Schizophrenia: manifestations, incidence and course in different cultures. A World Health Organization ten-country study. *Psychological medicine*, Suppl. 20.

Loranger AW et al. (1991) The WHO/ADAMHA International Pilot Study of Personality Disorders: background and purpose. *Journal of personality disorders*, 5: 296–306.

Robins LN et al. (1988) The Composite International Diagnostic Interview. *Archives of general psychiatry*, 45: 1069–1076.

Sartorius N et al. (1983) *Depressive disorders in different cultures*. Geneva, World Health Organization.

Sartorius N et al., eds. (1990) *Psychological disorders in general medical settings*. Berne, Huber.

WHO (1979) *Schizophrenia: an international follow-up study*. Chichester, Wiley.

WHO (1992a) *Global health situation and projections estimates*. Geneva, World Health Organization (unpublished document WHO/HST/92.1; available on request from Division of Epidemiological Surveillance and Health Situation and Trend Assessment, World Health Organization, 1211 Geneva 27, Switzerland).

WHO (1992b) *The ICD-10 Classification of Mental and Behavioural Disorders. Clinical descriptions and diagnostic guidelines*. Geneva, World Health Organization.

Wing JK et al. (1990) SCAN: Schedules for Clinical Assessment in Neuropsychiatry. *Archives of general psychiatry*, 47: 589–593.

Acknowledgements

The authors thank the following for reviewing the manuscript and for their valuable comments and suggestions: Dr W.W. Eaton, Department of Mental Hygiene, School of Hygiene and Public Health, Johns Hopkins University, Baltimore, MD, USA; Professor H. Häfner, Central Institute for Mental Health, Mannheim, Germany; Professor A. S. Henderson, Social Psychiatry Unit, National Health and Medical Research Council, Australian National University, Canberra, Australia; Professor A. Jablensky, University Department of Psychiatry and Behavioural Sciences, Royal Perth Hospital, Perth, Australia; Professor J. Leff, MRC Social and Community Psychiatry Unit, Institute of Psychiatry, London, England; Dr P. Munk-Jørgensen, Department of Psychiatric Demography, Institute of Basic Psychiatric Research, University of Aarhus, Denmark; and Professor J. Wing, Research Unit, Royal College of Psychiatrists, London, England. Thanks are also due to Professor N.C. Andreasen, Department of Psychiatry, University of Iowa Hospitals and Clinics, Iowa City, USA, and to Professor T. McGlashan, Yale Psychiatric Institute and Department of Psychiatry, Yale University, New Haven, USA, for their help with regard to the DSM-IV classification of schizophrenia; to Professor D. Goldberg, Institute of Psychiatry, London, England, for his comments on the epidemiology of schizophrenia in primary health care facilities; and to Professor N. Sartorius, formerly Director, Division of Mental Health, WHO, Geneva, for his valuable input and his continuous encouragement and support.

Acronyms and abbreviations used in this book

CIDI	Composite International Diagnostic Interview
CT	Computerized tomography
DIS	Diagnostic Interview Schedule
DOSMED	Determinants of Outcome of Severe Mental Disorders
DSM-III	*Diagnostic and Statistical Manual of Mental Disorders*, 3rd ed.
DSM-III-R	*Diagnostic and Statistical Manual of Mental Disorders*, 3rd ed. (revised)
DSM-IV	*Diagnostic and Statistical Manual of Mental Disorders*, 4th ed.
ECA	Epidemiologic Catchment Area
ICD-8	*Manual of the International Statistical Classification of Diseases, Injuries and Causes of Death. Eighth revision.*
ICD-9	*Manual of the International Statistical Classification of Diseases, Injuries and Causes of Death. Ninth revision.*
ICD-10	*International Statistical Classification of Diseases and Related Health Problems. Tenth revision.*
IQ	Intelligence quotient
MRI	Magnetic resonance imaging
NIMH	National Institute of Mental Health
PET	Positron emission tomography
PSE	Present State Examination
RDC	Research Diagnostic Criteria
SADS	Schedule for Affective Disorders and Schizophrenia
SCAN	Schedules for Clinical Assessment in Neuropsychiatry
SCID	Structured Clinical Interview for DSM-III-R
SD	Standard deviation

1
Introduction

Schizophrenia is a severe psychiatric disorder. The disease usually starts in adolescence or early adult life and often becomes chronic and disabling. The overall direct and indirect costs of the disorder are huge. According to one estimate, the treatment of schizophrenia in the United States, excluding indirect expenses, costs close to 0.5% of the gross national product (Gunderson & Mosher, 1975). The burden on the patient's family is heavy and both the patient and his or her relatives are often exposed to the stigma associated with the illness, sometimes over generations. Thus schizophrenia is a major public health problem.

The World Health Organization has focused special attention on schizophrenia, and has organized a number of studies aimed at improving understanding of the disorder and finding ways to deal with it. The WHO programme of collaborative clinical and epidemiological research on schizophrenia started in the late 1960s. Its first task was to develop a reliable methodology for comparative cross-cultural studies in different populations.

This monograph is a continuation of the previous work of the Organization in this area of enquiry, and aims to provide a broad overview of current knowledge about the epidemiology of schizophrenia. It starts with an examination of relevant diagnostic and methodological issues. Incidence and prevalence studies of schizophrenia are then reviewed, and similarities and differences in rates across different populations discussed. Risk factors for schizophrenia and temporal trends in the occurrence of the disorder are considered, with special emphasis on etiology. Finally, recommendations are made for future studies.

2
Diagnostic issues

Until the end of the eighteenth century, it was believed that all mental disorders were expressions of a single pathological entity, termed *Einheitspsychose* by the German alienists Zeller and Griesinger (Glatzel, 1990). Pinel was one of the earliest to recognize that mental disorders could be separated and classified according to their different features, distinguishing between dementia, idiocy, mania and melancholia. The French psychiatrist Morel was another important figure in this psychiatric school. In 1852, Morel gave the name *démence précoce* to a disorder leading initially to emotional withdrawal, odd mannerisms and self-neglect, and eventually to intellectual deterioration. Shortly after Morel, the German psychiatrists Hecker and Kahlbaum, in 1871 and 1883 respectively, described the syndromes of catatonia and hebephrenia.

The German psychiatrist, Emil Kraepelin, laid the foundations for the modern concept of schizophrenia. Studying patients admitted to mental hospitals in the late nineteenth century, he observed that certain types of insanity with an onset in early adult life and initially rather varied features, seemed to progress ultimately to a similar deteriorated condition. To accentuate the progressive deterioration of mental abilities, of emotional responses and of the integrity of the personality which he saw as central to this condition, Kraepelin termed it "dementia praecox" (dementia of early life). In 1896, in the fifth edition of his textbook, he suggested that three conditions, previously regarded as separate, were in fact subtypes of this single disease entity, which he distinguished from manic–depressive illness (Sass, 1987). The three conditions were hebephrenia, marked by aimless, disorganized and incongruous behaviour; catatonia, in which the individual might be negativistic, motionless or even stuporose, or, at other times, extremely agitated and incoherent; and, finally, dementia paranoides, in which delusions of persecution and grandeur were predominant. Kraepelin regarded dementia praecox as a condition characterized by a deteriorating, inevitably negative course and outcome, even though some 12% of his patients recovered more or less completely.

A few years later, the Swiss psychiatrist Eugen Bleuler made important contributions to the concept of the disorder. In 1908, he proposed the name "schizophrenia" to denote a splitting of psychic functions which he considered to be of paramount importance. He made a distinction between fundamental and accessory symptoms: the former included disturbances of thought associations, abnormal emotional reactions and a disturbance of volition. Accessory symptoms included hallucinations, delusions, catatonia, and abnormal and incomprehensible behaviour. Ambivalence and a new concept which Bleuler named "autism"—living in a fantasy world—were important features in his clinical description of the illness. In 1911, Bleuler published a monograph in which he emphasized that schizophrenia was a group of disorders rather than a single entity. He accepted Kraepelin's original three subgroups and added a fourth: simple schizophrenia. Bleuler's view of outcome in schizophrenia was substantially less pessimistic than that of Kraepelin, and he contended that, although full recovery from the disease was a rare occurrence, far-reaching improvement was common. Whereas Kraepelin emphasized the phenomenology of the disorder, Bleuler was more interpretative and gave special emphasis to the meaning of the symptoms (Bland & Kolada, 1988). Neither author, however, despite their detailed investigations, provided clear-cut diagnostic criteria for the condition.

After Bleuler, the German psychiatrist Kurt Schneider (1959) identified a group of eleven symptoms which he believed were pathognomonic of schizophrenia, and were rarely found in other psychiatric disorders. He called them "first-rank symptoms" — "not because we think of them as basic disturbances, but because they have this special value in helping us to determine the diagnosis of schizophrenia ... Symptoms of first rank importance do not always have to be present for a diagnosis to be made" (Schneider, 1959). Schneider's first-rank symptoms included hearing one's thoughts spoken aloud, auditory hallucinations that comment on one's behaviour, thought withdrawal or insertion, thought broadcasting and the feeling that one's actions are influenced by external agents. Schneider also identified a subset of symptoms which he called "second-rank symptoms"; they include other types of hallucinations, perplexity, sudden delusional ideas, depressive or euphoric mood changes and emotional blunting. He argued that schizophrenia can be diagnosed on the basis of the second-rank symptoms alone if they are sufficient in number.

The first-rank symptoms proposed by Schneider narrowed the concept of schizophrenia and have retained a crucial role in subsequent diagnostic systems: some of them are included in the ICD-10 and DSM-III diagnostic criteria for schizophrenia. Despite the great importance that has been placed on first-rank symptoms for the diagnosis of schizophrenia, their frequency in patients with this diagnosis varies significantly. In 13 studies reviewed by Fenton et al. (1981), the prevalence of first-rank symptoms ranged from a low of 24% to a high of 72% with a median value of 51%. Wulff (1967) suggested that the prevalence of first-rank symptoms is lower in patients from developing countries. This view is supported by a prospective study in which 169 patients in Sri Lanka, assessed with the Present State Examination (PSE), were compared with patients from two developed countries (Chandrasena, 1987). In the WHO Study on the Determinants of Outcome of Severe Mental Disorders (DOSMED) (Jablensky et al., 1992), an average of 56% of the patients with a clinical diagnosis of schizophrenia in the different centres exhibited one or more of the first-rank symptoms; these symptoms defined a subpopulation of schizophrenic patients characterized by elevated scores on positive psychotic symptoms. These patients showed a greater similarity across cultures than the total study population.

The specificity of first-rank symptoms has been disputed because they can be found in other disorders, especially mania (Carpenter & Strauss, 1974; Pope & Lipinski, 1978; Taylor & Abrams, 1975). Among the first-rank symptoms, the least discriminating is the "third person" hallucination — a voice or voices referring to the subject in the third person (Mellor, 1982).

In the Scandinavian countries an important contribution to the diagnostic concept of schizophrenia came in the 1930s from the Norwegian psychiatrist, Langfeldt. He distinguished between a core group of "process" or "nuclear" schizophrenics, who demonstrated an insidious onset of illness and a deteriorating course, and a "reactive" group, who tended to show signs of better social functioning before becoming psychotic, to have a more acute onset, often precipitated by stress, and to display a better prognosis. Following Langfeldt, reactive psychoses have been separated from "true" schizophrenia in Scandinavian psychiatric terminology and named "schizophreniform psychoses".

In France, one feature of the diagnostic tradition for schizophrenia has been the narrowing of the diagnosis and a corresponding increase in the number of nonschizophrenic delusional states (Pichot, 1990). The purpose of this differentiation is to emphasize the importance of a deteriorating course in making a diagnosis of "true" schizophrenia. A recent study (van Os et al., 1993) confirmed that psychiatrists in France and the United Kingdom use different diagnostic criteria. Responses to a questionnaire revealed that French psychiatrists are reluctant to diagnose schizophrenia in patients over 45 years of age. Despite the narrowing of the diagnosis to exclude good-prognosis or older cases, however, the French diagnosis of schizophrenia appears overall to be broader than in the United Kingdom. French psychiatrists use a Bleulerian psychoanalytic diagnostic approach which encompasses a variety of chronic states that would be excluded in the United Kingdom for lack of specific symptoms. They recognize, for example, a "pseudopsychopathic" subtype of schizophrenia. The current French approach is in many ways reminiscent of American diagnostic practices prior to the introduction of standardized criteria in the 1970s (van Os et al., 1993).

In the United States of America from 1950 until the mid-1970s, psychiatrists paid little attention to the issue of course in diagnosing schizophrenia and emphasized instead the presence of supposedly schizophrenic symptoms and defects. The result was an over-inclusive pattern of diagnosis for schizophrenia in comparison with European approaches. American psychiatrists referred mainly, in their diagnostic practice, to the Bleulerian "four As": disturbances of association between thoughts, disturbances of affect, autism, and morbid ambivalence.

The differences that existed between national diagnostic systems for schizophrenia, and in particular between the American and the European approaches, were clearly demonstrated in the 1960s by an international research project carried out in New York and London (Cooper et al., 1972). The study, which was stimulated by the work of Morton Kramer (Kramer, 1969; Kramer et al., 1961), examined hundreds of patients admitted to hospitals in these two cities and noted their hospital diagnoses. It was found that American psychiatrists were about twice as likely as the research team to diagnose schizophrenia, four times less likely to diagnose psychotic depression and ten times less likely to label a psychotic patient as suffering from mania. The diagnoses given by the psychiatrists working in London hospitals, as might be expected, were very close to those of the project psychiatrists (who were using a British diagnostic approach). Plainly, at that time, American psychiatrists were labelling as schizophrenic patients who would have been considered manic–depressive in the United Kingdom and in other European countries.

The problem of diagnostic variation between countries can be seen in broader cross-cultural perspective in the findings of the International Pilot Study of Schizophrenia (WHO, 1973, 1979). Using a standardized assessment (the Present State Examination, 9th edition) and diagnostic approach (based on ICD-8 and incorporated in the CATEGO computer program), the project evaluated the symptoms of psychotic patients admitted to treatment in nine centres in developed and developing countries—China (Province of Taiwan), Colombia, Czechoslovakia, Denmark, India, Nigeria, the United Kingdom, the United States and the USSR. Comparing the diagnoses made by the local hospital psychiatrists with the uniform research method, the project revealed that the diagnosis of psychosis in general, and schizophrenia in particular, was reasonably similar in the European and developing country centres. On the other hand, the Soviet and American diagnostic approaches were very different from those of the other centres. A large proportion of the patients who were labelled schizophrenic by psychiatrists in Moscow and Washington did not meet the research definition and would have been diagnosed as suffering from manic–depressive psychosis or a neurosis elsewhere in the world. The study confirmed that the diagnosis of schizophrenia was made differently in Europe than in the United States. In Europe, psychiatrists tended to use the diagnosis cautiously to refer to a small subset of patients with hallucinations and delusions not explicable in terms of affective disturbances during the first attack. In the United States, at that time, and to some extent in the USSR, the concept of schizophrenia traditionally included anyone with any type of hallucination or delusion, or with odd or incomprehensible behaviour.

The diagnostic approaches of American psychiatrists changed suddenly and radically in the mid-1970s. Much greater attention was paid to discriminating manic–depressive illness from schizophrenia and within a few years, different operational criteria for the diagnosis of schizophrenia appeared. In 1972, Feighner and associates published their diagnostic criteria based on patient, family and follow-up studies, while Astrachan and co-workers (1972) tried to devise a reliable checklist for making such diagnoses. Later developments included the Research Diagnostic Criteria (RDC) (Spitzer et al., 1977) and finally, in 1980, the third edition of the Diagnostic and Statistical Manual of Mental Disorders (DSM-III) (American Psychiatric Association, 1980).

As Andreasen & Flaum (1991) point out, the introduction of the new criteria represented an attempt to reverse the previous trend and to narrow the diagnostic criteria, essentially by two means: by introducing a six-month duration criterion, and by giving prominence to florid or positive symptoms with correspondingly less importance being given to deficit, negative (or "Bleulerian") symptoms.

2.1 Relevance of diagnostic issues for epidemiological research

The diagnostic issues discussed above are of critical importance for epidemiological research because changing the classification and diagnostic criteria for schizophrenia can significantly affect the prevalence of the disorder detected in community studies or treated samples. The differences between the various diagnostic systems are a result of the choice of symptom criteria, the structure of diagnostic algorithms, the duration criteria and the evaluation of affective symptoms. There are more than ten comparative studies using over a dozen diagnostic definitions of schizophrenia, showing that detected rates of the disorder depend on the diagnostic criteria adopted (Sass, 1987). In one of the most important of these studies, Endicott et al. (1982) compared the joint frequencies and reliabilities of six sets of diagnostic criteria (New Haven, Carpenter, Feighner, Taylor & Abrams, DSM-III and RDC) in a sample of 108 patients. The six systems were comparable in terms of reliability but the proportion of cases diagnosed as schizophrenia ranged between 4% and 26% depending on the diagnostic system, with RDC, DSM-III and Carpenter criteria being close to one another. The main reasons for the differences were related to (a) the criteria for exclusion of patients with affective disorders, (b) the duration criterion adopted, and (c) the degree of specificity of each item (for example, "hallucinations" versus "hallucinations of two or more voices conversing"). In another study, Brockington et al. (1978), comparing different sets of diagnostic criteria, found that the rate of schizophrenia in a series of 119 patients on first admission for psychiatric care varied between 3.4% and 38% depending on the criteria. RDC, CATEGO, Carpenter and Langfeldt's criteria showed good concordance.

The critical importance of the diagnostic criteria for the rate of schizophrenia found in community epidemiological studies has been clearly demonstrated by Helzer (1988). Using data from the St Louis site of the Epidemiologic Catchment Area (ECA) study, the author showed that a fivefold difference in the prevalence estimates was found when the Feighner, RDC and DSM-III criteria were applied to the same data set. This fivefold difference was of the same magnitude as that found by Dunham (1965) in his review of prevalence rates of schizophrenia in various European and North American countries. Thus differences of such a magnitude could be entirely related to the definitions used.

Other studies have demonstrated that a change in diagnostic habits can explain apparent variations over time in rates of schizophrenia among psychiatric patients. Kuriansky et al. (1974) found that 77% of patients admitted to the New York State Psychiatric Institute during the late 1940s and early 1950s were diagnosed as schizophrenic, compared with fewer than 28% of the admissions to the same hospital during the 1930s. Re-examination of the clinical data in the hospital records and rediagnosis of the cases indicated that the psychiatrists in the later period used a broader definition of schizophrenia. A survey carried out in one of the largest university-affiliated psychiatric hospitals in the USA (Loranger, 1990) compared the diagnoses given to 5143 patients in the last five years of the DSM-II era (1975–79) with those given in the first five years of the DSM-III era (1981–85) (5771 patients), and found a marked decrease in the diagnosis of schizophrenia, from 25% to 13%, together with an increase in the diagnosis of personality disorders and affective disorders. Many of the cases diagnosed as schizophreniform, atypical psychosis, reactive psychosis, and schizotypal personality disorder according to DSM-III criteria would have been diagnosed as schizophrenia with the DSM-II. However, all of these new categories combined accounted for only 5.3% of the total DSM-III sample and explain less than half the decline in the diagnosis of schizophrenia. The large increase in the diagnosis of affective disorders appears to have been the primary reason for the decrease in schizophrenia diagnoses. Unipolar depression rose from 15% to 25%, and bipolar disorder rose from 7% to 11%. The study confirms the previously noted tendency for American psychiatrists in the pre-DSM-III era to diagnose schizophrenia in cases where European psychiatrists would have made a diagnosis of affective disorder.

In another study, data on discharge diagnoses from 1972 to 1988 were gathered from six North American psychiatric teaching hospitals, and rates for schizophrenia and major mood disorders were evaluated (Stoll et al., 1993). Large reciprocal shifts in the frequencies of diagnoses of schizophrenia and major affective disorders were found. Beginning in the early 1970s, a gradual increase in the frequency of diagnoses of major affective disorders at all sites was accompanied by a corresponding decrease in diagnoses of schizophrenia at five of the six centres. Schizophrenia diagnoses decreased from a peak of 27% in 1976 to 9% in 1989 (a threefold decrease), while diagnoses of major affective disorders rose from a low of 10% in 1972 to 44% in 1990 (a fourfold increase). Among the reasons for this substantial shift, the authors include the narrowing in the DSM-III definition of schizophrenia and broadening in the category of major affective disorders.

2.2 ICD-10 classification of schizophrenia

Table 1 lists the group of schizophrenic disorders as classified by ICD-10, DSM-III-R (American Psychiatric Association, 1987) and DSM-IV (American Psychiatric Association, 1994). Annex 1 shows the ICD-10 clinical descriptions and diagnostic guidelines for the disorder.

A number of diagnostic issues in the ICD-10 classification of schizophrenic disorders merit comment. First, the group of schizophrenia, schizotypal states and delusional disorders (F20–F29) has been expanded by the introduction of new categories such as undifferentiated schizophrenia, post-schizophrenic

Table 1

Classification of schizophrenia and schizophrenia-like disorders in ICD-10, DSM-III-R and DSM-IV

ICD-10	DSM-III-R	DSM-IV
Schizophrenia	**Schizophrenia**	**Schizophrenia**
Paranoid	Paranoid	Paranoid
Hebephrenic	Disorganized	Disorganized
Catatonic	Catatonic	Catatonic
Undifferentiated	Undifferentiated	Undifferentiated
Residual	Residual	Residual
Post-schizophrenic depression		Postpsychotic depression of schizophrenia
Simple		Simple deterioration disorder (simple schizophrenia)
Other schizophrenia		
Schizophrenia, unspecified		
Schizotypal disorder		
Persistent delusional disorder	**Delusional (paranoid) disorder**	**Delusional disorder**
Acute and transient psychotic disorder		
Acute polymorphic psychotic disorder without symptoms of schizophrenia		
Acute polymorphic psychotic disorder with symptoms of schizophrenia	**Brief reactive psychosis**	**Brief psychotic disorder**
Acute schizophrenia-like psychotic disorder	**Schizophreniform disorder**	**Schizophreniform disorder**
Other acute predominantly delusional psychotic disorders		
Other acute and transient psychotic disorders		
Acute and transient psychotic disorders unspecified		
Induced delusional disorder	**Induced psychotic disorder**	**Induced psychotic disorder**
Schizoaffective disorders	**Schizoaffective disorders**	**Schizoaffective disorder**
Other nonorganic psychotic disorders		
		Secondary psychotic disorder due to a general medical condition
		– with delusions
		– with hallucinations
		Substance-induced psychotic disorder
Unspecified nonorganic psychoses	**Psychotic disorder not otherwise specified**	**Psychotic disorder not otherwise specified**

depression and schizotypal disorder. Schizotypal states are of two types, namely schizotypal disorder and simple schizophrenia; the latter refers to a disorder with an insidious development of negative symptoms without delusions or hallucinations. After long debate, it was determined that schizoaffective disorders (F25), as defined in the ICD-10, should be placed in the same group as schizophrenia, rather than with affective disorders (F30–F39). For a diagnosis of schizoaffective disorder at least one typically schizophrenic symptom must be present with affective symptoms during the same episode.

An important issue is the duration of symptoms required to distinguish schizophrenia from acute and transient psychotic disorders (F23). Several authors have stressed the high frequency of these disorders in developing countries and the need to classify them adequately (Wig & Parhee, 1989). In ICD-10 the diagnosis of schizophrenia requires the presence of typical delusions, hallucinations or other symptoms for a minimum of one month. There are strong clinical traditions in several countries, based upon descriptive though not epidemiological studies, suggesting that Kraepelin's dementia praecox and Bleuler's schizophrenias are distinct from acute psychoses with abrupt onset, a short course of a few weeks or days, and a favourable outcome. Terms such as *bouffée délirante*, psychogenic psychosis, schizophreniform psychosis, cycloid psychosis and brief reactive psychosis indicate the widespread opinion that this form of psychosis should be considered as distinct from schizophrenia. Opinions and evidence vary as to whether these disorders are usually or always associated with acute psychological stress and whether they may occur with transient but typical schizophrenic symptoms. (*Bouffée délirante*, at least, was originally described as not usually being associated with an obvious psychological precipitant.) In the present state of knowledge about schizophrenia and these more acute disorders, it was considered that the best option would be to allow sufficient time for the disorder to appear, be recognized and largely subside before considering a diagnosis of schizophrenia. Most clinical reports and authorities suggest that the large majority of patients with acute transient psychoses have an onset of psychotic symptoms over a few days, at most two weeks, and that many recover with or without medication within 2–3 weeks. It seemed appropriate, therefore, to specify at least one month of clear and typical schizophrenic symptoms before the disorder can be diagnosed as schizophrenia.

The adoption of a criterion of only one month's duration of typical psychotic symptoms for the diagnosis of schizophrenia rejects the assumption that schizophrenia must be of comparatively long duration. A duration of six months has been adopted in several national classifications, but for the ICD-10 it was felt that there are no advantages in restricting the diagnosis of schizophrenia in this way. In two WHO studies—the International Pilot Study of Schizophrenia and the Determinants of Outcome of Severe Mental Disorders—a substantial proportion of patients had clear and typical schizophrenic symptoms for more than one month but less than six months, and made good if not complete recoveries from the disorder. It therefore seemed appropriate to avoid assumptions about chronicity and regard schizophrenia as a descriptive term for a syndrome that has a variety of causes (many of which are still unknown) and a variety of outcomes, depending upon the balance of genetic, physical, social and cultural influences.

The term "schizophreniform" has not been used for a defined disorder in the ICD-10 classification. This is because it has been applied to several different

9

clinical concepts over the past few decades, and associated with a variety of characteristics such as acute onset, relatively brief duration, atypical symptoms or mixtures of symptoms, and comparatively good outcome. There is, as yet, no evidence in favour of a preferred choice of usage, so the case for its inclusion as a diagnostic term was considered to be weak. The need for an intermediate category of this type, moreover, was removed by the inclusion of the category of acute and transient psychotic disorders (F23) and its subdivisions, together with the requirement for one month of psychotic symptoms for a diagnosis of schizophrenia.

During the preparation of ICD-10, a large number of clinical field trials were conducted to establish inter-rater reliability. Two methods of estimating inter-rater reliability were calculated: pair-wise agreement rates and kappa coefficients (Sartorius et al., 1993). A total of 557 clinicians at 95 clinical centres in 33 different countries participated in the joint assessment phase of the draft of ICD-10. They made 9012 assessments for 2385 patients of widely varying ages. Male and female patients were represented approximately equally in the field trials.

For the group schizophrenia, schizotypal and delusional disorders (F20–F29), the kappa coefficient was satisfactory (0.82). The agreement for diagnoses at the three-character category level varied according to the category, with a high value for schizophrenia (0.81) and lower values for other diagnoses (e.g. 0.46 for schizotypal states). (By comparison, we may note that in a review of prior studies reporting the reliability of a clinical diagnosis of schizophrenia, Spitzer & Fleiss (1974) found the average kappa coefficient to be no better than 0.57.) For the four-character categories of schizophrenic disorders, the kappa values were also variable, with acceptable values for paranoid schizophrenia (0.73) and hebephrenic schizophrenia (0.65), and a low value for undifferentiated schizophrenia (0.44).

For each diagnostic assessment, clinicians were also asked to make a rating on the following scales: (a) goodness of fit of the diagnostic category with the case observed, (b) confidence in use of diagnosis, (c) ease or difficulty of diagnosis, and (d) adequacy of clinical description and diagnostic guidelines. The main diagnostic problems were found to be with schizotypal disorder, acute schizophrenia-like disorder and other acute psychotic disorders, while the specific ICD-10 categories of schizophrenia were rated as satisfactory.

2.3   DSM-III-R and DSM-IV classifications of schizophrenia

DSM-III-R classifies schizophrenia according to the symptoms of the acute phase and the course of the illness. A course requirement for the diagnosis is the presence of continuous signs of disturbance for at least six months. The acute symptoms (criterion A) are divided into three sets. The first set includes delusions, hallucinations, incoherence or marked loosening of associations, catatonic behaviour, and flat or inappropriate affect. The second set consists of "bizarre" delusions which would seem implausible to other members of the same cultural group (e.g. thought-broadcasting or being controlled by a dead person). The third set consists of special kinds of auditory hallucinations. Thus, for a diagnosis of schizophrenia according to DSM-III-R criteria, the presence of positive psychotic symptoms (delusions, hallucinations, or thought disorder) is required.

Compared with the DSM-III, the DSM-III-R criteria for schizophrenia were simplified through a reduction of the subcategories in criterion A from six items to three. The diagnosis remained complex, however, as the clinician had to assess the presence of at least 12 different signs and symptoms. While DSM-III contained no duration requirement for the acute symptoms in criterion A, DSM-III-R required the presence of one or more such symptoms for at least one week. The requirement that affective disorder should be excluded was moved from a subsidiary position in DSM-III to a central position in DSM-III-R, where it is equal in importance with delusions, hallucinations, thought disorder, and catatonic behaviour. Among the prodromal or residual symptoms was included a marked lack of initiative, interest or energy. The B criterion, concerning deterioration in functioning was broadened in DSM-III-R to include failure to achieve expected level of social development. The age criterion for schizophrenia ("onset of prodromal or active phase of illness before age 45") was eliminated from DSM-III-R. As Andreasen & Flaum (1991) pointed out, the net effect of these changes appeared to be a further narrowing of the definition of schizophrenia in DSM-III-R. Other changes were made to the diagnostic criteria for delusional (paranoid) disorders, brief reactive psychosis, schizophreniform disorder and schizoaffective disorder (Kendler et al., 1989).

The new DSM-IV requires one month of active A criterion symptoms, like ICD-10 and unlike the one week required by DSM-III-R. On the other hand, DSM-IV, like DSM-III-R, requires a total duration of 6 months, at least one month of active symptoms and at most 5 months of negative and attenuated positive symptoms (detailed prodromal and residual symptoms are no longer specified). The DSM-IV criteria contain two positive symptoms (hallucinations and delusions) and one negative symptom group (affective flattening, alogia, avolition). Finally, DSM-IV excludes schizophrenia in the presence of manic or depressive moods that are substantially longer in duration than the psychotic symptoms.

2.4 Similarities and dissimilarities between ICD-10, DSM-III-R and DSM-IV

The main differences between ICD-10 and DSM-III-R in the classification of schizophrenia are the duration criterion (one month for ICD-10 compared with six months for DSM-III-R) and the greater weight given in the ICD-10 to Schneiderian first-rank symptoms. Negative symptoms are emphasized more in the ICD-10, because they are spelt out and can be used for the diagnosis of the disorder if they are present in conjunction with thought disorder (e.g. irrelevant speech). The greater importance given in ICD-10 to first-rank symptoms has the effect of narrowing the diagnosis, while the shorter duration requirement, the reliance on negative symptoms and the inclusion of simple schizophrenia tend to increase the number of patients embraced by the category of schizophrenia.

The definition of schizoaffective disorder in ICD-10 differs from that in DSM-III-R in that it adopts an essentially cross-sectional approach and requires the simultaneous presence of psychotic and affective symptoms. There are other notable differences with respect to the classification of other schizophrenia-like disorders. As may be seen in Table 1, ICD-10 recognizes nine subtypes of schizophrenia, including post-schizophrenic depression. For five of the subtypes there is a direct correspondence between ICD-10, DSM-III-R, and DSM-IV. For one of these, the ICD-10 has used a different term ("hebephrenic" as opposed to "disorganized" in the DSM-III-R and DSM-IV). Two other subtypes included in ICD-10 are not in the DSM-III-R classification (post-schizophrenic depression and simple schizophrenia), but are present in DSM-IV. Finally, two ICD-10 categories ("other schizophrenia" and "schizophrenia, unspecified") are not included in either of the American diagnostic systems.

A recent literature review analysed available evidence concerning the validity of the current subtypes of schizophrenia (McGlashan & Fenton, 1991). There are few relevant studies, but the data support the validity of the paranoid, hebephrenic, undifferentiated and residual subtypes. Catatonic schizophrenia has been least studied, perhaps owing to the rarity of this subtype in the developed world (McGlashan & Fenton, 1991). Because of the historical prominence of simple schizophrenia and the growing importance of deficit processes in schizophrenia, the authors of the review advocated the reintroduction of this subtype in DSM-IV (which has, in fact, taken place).

As regards DSM-IV, positive and negative symptoms are presented in a more generic and less detailed fashion than in either DSM-III-R or ICD-10, but cover the same phenomenological territory. Negative symptoms have received greater prominence in DSM-IV than in DSM-III-R. DSM-IV retains the special significance of bizarre delusions and Schneiderian hallucinations, which have been part of both DSM-III-R and ICD-10. Deterioration of functioning continues to be a criterion in DSM-IV as in DSM-III-R, unlike ICD-10 which has no corresponding requirement.

One study has compared the reliability and ease of use of ICD-10 (clinical and research versions) and DSM-III-R among a small sample of psychiatrists working in pairs to diagnose 60 patients (Mellsop et al., 1991). All three systems showed similar, high inter-rater and inter-system agreement for the general diagnostic categories of schizophrenia but not for subtypes, such as paranoid or hebephrenic schizophrenia. The compatibility between ICD-10 and DSM-III-R for schizophrenia was much closer than that between ICD-8 and DSM-III. It is likely, therefore, that the findings of epidemiological studies carried out using the latest diagnostic systems will be more comparable than those resulting from the earlier ones.

Copeland et al. (1991) caution that standardized diagnostic criteria are useless if investigators use them in an incomplete or variable manner. Accordingly, diagnostic criteria need to be accompanied by standardized instruments and algorithms for their consistent implementation, if full benefit is to be gained from them.

2.5 Assessment methods

As described above, there has been a movement, over the years, towards establishing and testing specific operational criteria for the diagnosis of schizophrenia. This has made it possible to reduce one of the two main sources of variability among diagnosticians, namely *criterion variance*. This term applies to differences in the formal, but unstated, inclusion and exclusion criteria that clinicians use in categorizing patient data to make psychiatric diagnoses. It is evident, however, that the development of specific criteria for making diagnoses does not ensure that clinicians will elicit and evaluate information in a uniform manner. This problem leads to the second main form of diagnostic variability, namely *information variance*. In order to reduce information variance, detailed interview schedules have been developed. Among the first of these were the Present State Examination (PSE) based on the ICD-8 criteria (Wing et al., 1974), the Renard Diagnostic Interview (Helzer et al., 1981) based on Feighner criteria, and the Schedule for Affective Disorders and Schizophrenia (SADS) (Spitzer & Endicott, 1978) based on the RDC.

Recent developments in this area include the Diagnostic Interview Schedule (DIS), the Structured Clinical Interview for DSM-III-R (SCID), the Composite International Diagnostic Interview (CIDI), the Schedules for Clinical Assessment in Neuropsychiatry (SCAN), and the Royal Park Multi-diagnostic Instrument for Psychosis (McGorry et al., 1990). These instruments will be reviewed briefly.

The DIS (Robins et al., 1981) was originally developed for the Epidemiologic Catchment Area (ECA) study. The instrument, which covers 43 DSM-III categories, is a highly structured interview, with every question written out in full to be read verbatim to the respondent. It can be used by either lay examiners or clinicians, and provides for an assessment of the lifetime history of psychiatric disturbance, including the age at each positive diagnosis, the age at most recent difficulty, and the duration of the longest episode. As pointed out in section 3.1.1, the validity of the DIS in schizophrenia in community studies is weak (Anthony et al., 1985; Helzer et al., 1985). Many of those identified by the DIS as schizophrenic do not, in fact, suffer from the illness but are people with relatively good functioning who report (and perhaps exaggerate) private bizarre experiences. It is also questionable whether an interview such as the DIS can successfully identify those who suffer from an illness of which an important feature is lack of insight. The DIS fails, not so much in the reporting of hallucinations and delusions, but more in the reporting of associated deterioration in functioning, and in observation of behaviour (Eaton et al., 1991). The DIS now includes DSM-III-R criteria, as well as symptom onset and recency: this change, while improving the general utility of the instrument, does little to alleviate its flaws for use in epidemiological studies of schizophrenia.

Another assessment instrument based on DSM-III is the SCID (Spitzer & Williams, 1985). The SCID differs from the DIS in that it is a semi-structured interview; thus, examiners need considerable clinical experience and some familiarity with DSM-III in order to use the instrument correctly. In consequence, the SCID is more appropriate than the DIS for the detection of serious disorders such as schizophrenia, which requires some direct observation. In addition, the SCID uses summary and screening questions, which allow the interviewer to skip irrelevant sections of the instrument.

The CIDI and the SCAN were devised recently in the framework of a large international collaborative project (Pull & Wittchen, 1991; Robins et al., 1988; Wing et al., 1990). These two instruments have different aims: the CIDI is intended primarily for surveys in the general population while the SCAN is meant for studies of clinical samples. The CIDI is a clear, highly structured, easily used interview schedule; it is based on the DIS, and has adopted certain features of the PSE-9. It can be administered by non-clinicians as well as by clinicians. The interview questions are fully spelt out and "closed ended" (i.e. answerable by a number or by choosing among predetermined alternatives); the answers do not need to be interpreted by the interviewer. CIDI is divided into 15 sections, of which one is for schizophrenia and other psychotic disorders. It allows diagnoses on a lifetime as well as on a cross-sectional basis. The average duration of the interview with respondents from the general population is about 75 minutes; with psychiatric patients it takes considerably longer. The core version of the CIDI is currently available in 16 languages.

Field trials with the CIDI have been conducted in 18 centres around the world to test the feasibility and reliability of the instrument in different cultures and settings as well as to test the inter-rater agreement for the different questions. A total of 557 subjects were interviewed in a variety of settings ranging from specialized psychiatric inpatient and outpatient units to general practice settings, and were rated by an interviewer and an observer (Wittchen et al., 1991). The kappa values for inter-rater reliability between centres were excellent for schizophrenia (0.91).

The SCAN is a network of instruments designed with the aim of developing a comprehensive procedure for clinical examination that is capable of classifying subjects according to categories of ICD-10 and DSM-III-R. Basically, SCAN is a continuation of the PSE tradition: it includes as a core component the PSE-10, and all the components of the interview are processed by a computer program, CATEGO 5. The instrument structures the clinical examination and provides ratings of each symptom and sign; although it is substantially structured, it retains the features of a clinical interview. It can be used in its full form only by professionals experienced in diagnostic assessment: the interviewer should have an understanding of basic psychopathology in terms of phenomenology, and should know how to conduct a clinical interview using probes to cross-examine for the presence of defined symptoms. The instrument is subdivided into two parts: part I is concerned with neurotic symptoms and eating and substance abuse disorders, together with a screen for part II; part II covers psychotic and cognitive disorders, and abnormalities of behaviour, affect and speech. The time span covered by the diagnostic assessment can vary, although the major focus of attention is functioning in the past month. The administration of the full SCAN usually takes about two hours. As with previous editions of the PSE, the severity of individual symptoms is rated and this can be used to generate the so-called "index of definition" i.e. the likelihood that the clinical picture is severe enough for the subject to be considered as suffering from a disorder. The core instruments of SCAN are currently available in 16 languages.

The Royal Park Multidiagnostic Instrument for Psychosis is a validity-oriented procedure recently developed for the assessment of acute psychotic episodes. It uses serial information and multiple information sources to construct a database of clinical information (McGorry et al., 1990). A number of sets of operational criteria, including 11 definitions of schizophrenia and several concepts of atypical, schizoaffective and affective psychoses, are simultaneously applied to this database to produce a diagnostic profile for each patient that can be linked to other variables.

The introduction of these standardized assessment methods for the diagnosis of schizophrenia represents a major step forward in epidemiological research and is expected to lead to a higher rate of reliability in the assessment process.

2.6 Case-finding methods

Four principal methods of case-finding may be used in epidemiological research on schizophrenia.

One method is the community survey, in which every accessible member of a community, or a selected sample of respondents from that community, is interviewed. This approach has proved feasible for small communities in geographically limited areas, but for large populations some sort of stratified or random sampling is required. In fact, given the low occurrence rate of schizophrenia, its epidemiological study requires very large population samples in order to detect a sufficient number of cases.

Another approach uses a psychiatric case register of patients and their contacts with treatment services. It was thought, until recently, that almost all patients suffering from a schizophrenic disorder in the developed world would sooner or later come to clinical attention and therefore be recorded in a local case register. Recent studies have cast doubt on this assumption, which may have become less valid in recent years as the community treatment of mental illness has become more common. This case-finding approach clearly depends on a well-functioning case register—an expensive mechanism which is available in few communities.

A third strategy relies on the identification of selected key informants, known in the community for having wide social contacts and an intimate knowledge of the culture. This approach has been applied in several epidemiological studies in the developing world, but has limitations in the complex and more anonymous setting of industrial societies.

A fourth approach relies on information available at various treatment facilities, including psychiatric hospitals, community mental health centres, general hospitals, general practitioners' clinics etc. The main limitations of this approach are (a) the under-representation of people with the disorder who do not have contact with treatment centres, and (b) a skewed reporting of cases with clinical or sociodemographic characteristics that are not representative of all the persons with the disorder in the community.

Any case-finding approach has its strengths and limitations. A comprehensive strategy for epidemiological research may require a combination of different approaches.

3

Epidemiology of schizophrenia

3.1 Incidence studies

Some authors, including Torrey (1980), have argued that the rate of occurrence of schizophrenia is very different in different settings; others, such as Leff (1988), argue that it is remarkably similar in frequency. The discrepancy in opinion is traceable, in large part, to methodological problems in the estimation of rates of incidence and prevalence of the disorder. Prevalence data are a reflection not only of the occurrence of a condition but also of its duration (which is affected by life expectancy). This can be expressed by Kramer's (1957) formula:

prevalence (P) = incidence (I) × duration (D).

In addition, we need to take into account that migration is an additional and important variable affecting the relationship between prevalence and incidence. Whereas prevalence statistics are of some value in planning the delivery of services, incidence rates are a more precise indicator of the occurrence of an illness and are more useful in the development of etiological theories.

In determining the incidence rate, the best way to obtain an accurate count of cases is to conduct a door-to-door survey, and for skilled clinicians to interview suspected cases in order to arrive at a diagnosis according to standardized criteria and to determine the date of onset of the condition. As mentioned earlier, in the case of illnesses with a low frequency of occurrence, such as schizophrenia, the population that would have to be surveyed to determine the incidence rate is so large that a door-to-door survey is impractical. Incidence data are generally derived, therefore, by counting the new cases seen at treatment facilities within a population over a given period of time (treated incidence rate). The accuracy of this approach depends on how many cases enter treatment and how many treatment facilities and practitioners are included in the case-finding process. Ideally, private practitioners and psychiatric wards of general hospitals should be included, but in many studies these sources are not surveyed. Inadequacies of case-finding are a major source of bias and contribute to the observed variation in incidence rates for schizophrenia.

Another source of variation in reported rates is the wide range of diagnostic approaches used by practitioners in different parts of the world and at different times. In order to reduce this source of confusion, the incidence data in the studies listed in Table 2 have been categorized as "narrow" (meaning the core schizophrenic syndrome defined by the CATEGO S + category), "standard" (the usual clinical approach used throughout much of the world), and "broad" (the diagnostic approach used in the USA before the introduction of DSM-III in 1980 and which included most cases categorized elsewhere as mania or psychotic depression) (Cooper et al., 1972). Even within the standard category, there is a wide range of diagnostic approaches: some of these studies restrict the diagnosis to category 295 in ICD-9 (schizophrenic psychoses); others include disorders in category 297 (paranoid states) and some disorders in category 298 (nonorganic psychoses). The Scandinavian concept of schizophrenia tends to be restrictive and the Soviet concept broad, but both are included here in the "standard" diagnostic category.

The effect of diagnosis on the observed incidence rate is evident in the study by Ní Nualláin and co-workers (1987) in Ireland, in which use of the ICD diagnosis resulted in an incidence rate (0.37 per 1000) twice as great as that detected by the CATEGO S + category (0.17 per 1000). Similarly, in a survey by Giel et al. (1980) in the Netherlands, the incidence rate for schizophrenia (ICD category 295) (0.03 per 1000) was one-quarter of the rate when paranoid states (ICD category 297) and reactive and psychogenic psychoses (ICD categories 298.4 and 298.8) were included (0.11 per 1000).

An additional reason for variation in reported incidence rates is the difference in the proportion of the population that has reached the age of risk for schizophrenia. Developing countries, for example, tend to have a higher proportion of children in the population and, therefore, a smaller at-risk group. Many studies calculate incidence as the rate of occurrence in the at-risk age group. These age-corrected rates will be greater than those that are not corrected for age: the two rates are not comparable and are listed separately in Table 2.

Special factors, which will be discussed below, may explain the exceptionally high incidence figures emerging from the recent United States Epidemiologic Catchment Area (ECA) survey (Tien & Eaton, 1992) and presented in Table 2. Apart from this study the variation in the rates in Table 2 is relatively slight. The mean age-corrected incidence for schizophrenia, excluding very narrow and very broad diagnostic approaches and excluding the ECA data, is 0.24 per 1000, with a range of 0.07 to 0.52 per 1000 (standard deviation (SD) 0.11). The studies from which this mean is derived used a variety of age ranges, which increases the variation in incidence rates. The mean incidence of schizophrenia using the standard diagnostic approaches, without correction for age, is 0.21 per 1000 (range 0.05–0.56) (SD 0.14). When the diagnosis is limited to the restrictive CATEGO S + "core" schizophrenic syndrome and corrected for age, the range of incidence is narrower (0.07–0.17 per 1000; mean 0.11; SD 0.03). With age correction and narrow diagnostic criteria, therefore, there is little variation in the reported incidence of schizophrenia.

3.1.1 The NIMH Epidemiologic Catchment Area study

An unusually high incidence of schizophrenia and a high degree of variability were determined by the Epidemiologic Catchment Area (ECA) study, a recent prospective field survey of five communities in the United States, conducted by the National Institute of Mental Health. Analysing data collected on two occasions a year apart by trained non-clinician interviewers using the Diagnostic Interview Schedule (DIS) (see section 2.5), Tien & Eaton (1992) found an annual age-corrected incidence rate of schizophrenia of between 1.0 and 7.1 per 1000. These rates are up to 25 times higher than the mean incidence rates found in other studies using a standard diagnostic approach. Even without the data from Baltimore (the site with the highest rate), the combined annual incidence for the other four sites is 1.1 cases per 1000, which is higher than any previously determined figure.

The authors offer two possible explanations for the unusually high rates in the ECA study. A prospective community-based survey, they suggest, is able to detect people who have not been in touch with help agencies and would not be detected in clinically based studies. Previous ECA data have indicated that about half of the active cases of schizophrenia are not *currently* receiving treatment, but to remain undetected by a clinically based incidence study a case must *never* come in contact with the agencies in the survey. This explanation, therefore, accounts for less than a doubling of the observed incidence rate. In two other studies, moreover—the Lundby study (Hagnell et al., 1990) and a survey carried out in Madras by Rajkumar et al. (quoted by Eaton, 1991)—cases were detected irrespective of whether the individual had been in treatment or not, and yet the rates (0.24 and 0.58 per 1000 respectively) were substantially lower than those found in the ECA study.

The authors also suggest that the high incidence rate may be due to a high number of false-positive cases being detected during the second interview at the end of the one-year study period. The use of non-clinicians as interviewers could have led to a substantial number of false-positives or false-negatives. When compared with evaluation by psychiatrists using the Present State Examination, the DIS is more likely to produce false-negatives than false-positives (Tien & Eaton, 1992). In the detection of relatively rare illnesses such as schizophrenia, however, a bias in the assessment of cases will result in many more non-cases being rated as positive (since there are so many more non-cases) than true cases being rated as negative.

A very high, divergent incidence figure was reported in the ECA survey for Baltimore. When a subsample of 810 of the Baltimore subjects was submitted to clinical evaluation by psychiatrists (Anthony et al., 1985), high false-negative and false-positive rates were revealed. Only 16% of the cases diagnosed as schizophrenia by lay interviewers using the DIS were confirmed as schizophrenia by the psychiatrists; and only 21% of the cases diagnosed as schizophrenic by the psychiatrists were detected by the DIS interview. In one case, the DIS interviewer wrote marginal notes about a subject's bizarre behaviour, but there was no DIS coding item for the notes. In another instance,

Table 2
Incidence of schizophrenia

Authors	Country or area	Population	Sample	Case-finding method	Diagnostic assessment
Ödegaard (1946)	Norway	Entire country	All first admissions, 1926–35 ($n = 14\,231$)		Hospital diagnosis
Shepherd (1957)	UK	Buckinghamshire ($n = 271\,586$ in 1931) ($n = 364\,257$ in 1947)	First admissions, 1931–33 1945–47		Hospital diagnosis
Hollingshead & Redlich (1958)	USA	New Haven, CT ($n = 174\,000$)	All individuals in treatment, 6 month period	Census of hospitals, clinics, practitioners	Facility diagnosis & study rediagnosis
Norris (1959)	UK	Catchment area ($n = 1\,661\,000$)	All admissions, 1947–49	Record tracing, 2-year follow-up	
Jaco (1960)	USA	State of Texas ($n = 7.7$ million)	All first admissions, 1951–52 ($n = 2701$)	Hospital, clinic & practitioner records	
Pollack et al. (1964)	USA	LA, MD	First admissions, 1960–61	Census matching of patients from public, private mental hospitals, veterans administrations, general hospitals	Hospital diagnosis
Dunham (1965)	USA	Two districts of Detroit ($n = 118\,577$)	All first admissions, 1958	Screening of all psychiatric facilities	Facility diagnosis
Warthen et al. (1967)	USA	MD	First admissions, 1963	Case register, all facilities except private outpatient practice	Facility diagnosis

Age group for calculation of rate (years)	Incidence per 1000 population per year					
	Narrow diagnosis		Standard diagnosis		Broad diagnosis	
	Without age correction	With age correction	Without age correction	With age correction	Without age correction	With age correction
> 9				0.24		
			0.10			
			0.05			
> 14						0.30
			0.17			
> 14					0.35	0.49
					0.44	
					0.47	
> 14					0.59	0.77
					0.50	

Table 2 (cont.)

Authors	Country or area	Population	Sample	Case-finding method	Diagnostic assessment
Adelstein et al. (1968)	UK	Salford ($n = 150\,000$)	All contacts in inception episodes	Case register	Hospital diagnosis (ICD 295)
Walsh (1969)	Ireland	Dublin ($n = 720\,000$)	All first admissions ($n = 1427$)		Hospital diagnosis
Häfner & Reimann (1970)	Fed. Rep. of Germany	Mannheim ($n = 328\,106$)	First contacts, 1965	Case register, state & private hospitals, practitioners, welfare & help agencies	Facility diagnosis (ICD 295, 297, 298.3, 298.4)
Hailey et al. (1974)	UK	Camberwell			ICD 295
Hailey et al. (1974)	UK	Salford			ICD 295
Liebermann (1974)	USSR	Moscow ($n = 248\,000$)	All onsets, 1910–64	Dispensary register	Records, personal examination
Bland et al.	Canada	State of Alberta ($n = 662\,181$)	All first admissions, 1963	Provincial hospital records	DSM-III & ICD-8 diagnoses
Nielsen (1976)	Denmark	Samsö Island ($n = 6823$)	All service contacts, 1964	General practitioners' case register	Facility diagnosis
Helgason (1977)	Iceland	Entire country	All first treatment contacts, 1966–67	National case register & hospital & disability records	ICD-8 295
Krasik & Semin (1980)	USSR	Tomsk	First admissions, 1948–51 1959–61 1969–71	District mental hospital	Facility diagnosis

22

	Incidence per 1000 population per year					
Age group for calculation of rate (years)	Narrow diagnosis		Standard diagnosis		Broad diagnosis	
	Without age correction	With age correction	Without age correction	With age correction	Without age correction	With age correction
> 14				0.31		
> 9				0.52		
			0.54			
			0.14			
			0.11			
			0.20			
15–60			0.14	0.11		
			0.20			
> 14			0.27	0.40		
			0.08			
			0.14			
			0.23			

Table 2 (cont.)

Authors	Country or area	Population	Sample	Case-finding method	Diagnostic assessment
Babigian (1980)	USA	Monroe County, NY	First contacts, 1970	Case register, hospitals, clinics & practitioners	Facility diagnosis
Giel et al. (1980)	Netherlands	Groningen & Drenthe	First contacts, 1975	Case register	ICD-8 (295, 297, 298.4, 298.8, 298.9)
Shen (1981)	China	Haidan district, Beijing (n = 156 200)	All onsets, 1974–77	Screening of village population by "barefoot doctors"	Psychiatrists' diagnosis
Krupinski (1983)	Australia	Victoria	First contacts, 1980		
Bates & van Dam (1984)	Canada	Vancouver Island, coastal Indians	First admissions, 1975–83	Case register	Hospital diagnosis
Eagles & Whalley (1985)	UK	Scotland	First admissions, 1969 1978	Health service register	Hospital diagnosis ICD-8 (295)
Munk-Jørgensen (1986)	Denmark	Entire country	First admissions, 1970 1984	Case register	Facility diagnosis
Ní Nualláin et al. (1987)	Ireland	Rosscommon, Carlow, Westmeath (n = 150 000)	First contacts, 1974–77	Case register, psychiatric services, inpatient and outpatient	Clinical or research diagnosis CATEGO/ICD-9 (295,297) Research diagnosis CATEGO S +
Kaličanin (1987)	Yugoslavia	Belgrade			
Dilling et al. (1989)	Fed. Rep. of Germany	Upper Bavaria (n = 424 000)	First contacts, 1971	Case register, hospital, clinic & office practice	Facility diagnosis

	Incidence per 1000 population per year					
Age group for calcu-lation of rate (years)	Narrow diagnosis		Standard diagnosis		Broad diagnosis	
	Without age correction	With age correction	Without age correction	With age correction	Without age correction	With age correction
					0.69	0.94
15–44				0.11		
			0.11			
			0.18			
			0.10			
			0.20			
			0.12			
> 14						
				0.11		
				0.07		
15–64				0.37		
		0.17				
			0.22			
			0.48			

Table 2 (cont.)

Authors	Country or area	Population	Sample	Case-finding method	Diagnostic assessment
Folnegović et al. (1990)	Yugoslavia	Croatia	First admissions, 1965–84	Case register	ICD-7, ICD-8, ICD-9
Der et al. (1990)	UK	England	First admissions, 1970 1986	Health service register	Hospital diagnosis: schizophrenia, paranoia, schizoaffective disorder
Hagnell et al. (1990)	Sweden	Lundby	General population survey		
Rajkumar et al. (1991)	India	Madras	General population survey		
Bamrah et al. (1991)	UK	Salford (*n* = 91 552)	All first contacts, 1984	Case register, general practitioners	ICD-9 (295, 297)
Häfner & Gattaz (1991)	Fed. Rep. of Germany	Mannheim (*n* = 300 000)	First contacts, 1985	Case register, state & private hospitals, practitioners, help agencies	Facility diagnosis (ICD 295, 297, 298.3, 298.4)
Häfner & Gattaz (1991)	Fed. Rep. of Germany	Rhine-Neckar district (*n* = 1 488 205)	First admissions, 1989–90	10 hospitals	CATEGO S +
Häfner (1991)	Fed. Rep. of Germany	Rhine-Neckar district (*n* = 1 488 205)	First admissions, 1987–89 (*n* = 392)	10 hospitals	ICD (295, 297, 298.3, 298.4)
Jablensky et al. (1992)	Denmark	Aarhus	First contacts, 1978–80	All help agencies	CATEGO S + CATEGO S,P,O or clinical diagnosis

	Incidence per 1000 population per year					
Age group for calculation of rate (years)	Narrow diagnosis		Standard diagnosis		Broad diagnosis	
	Without age correction	With age correction	Without age correction	With age correction	Without age correction	With age correction
> 15			0.22	0.27		
				0.16		
				0.09		
			0.24			
> 15				0.58		
> 15				0.19		
			0.56			
15–54		0.09				
			0.13			
15–54		0.07		0.18		

Table 2 (cont.)

Authors	Country or area	Population	Sample	Case-finding method	Diagnostic assessment
Jablensky et al. (1992)	India	Chandigarh (rural)	First contacts, 1978–80	All help agencies	CATEGO S + CATEGO S,P,O or clinical diagnosis
Jablensky et al. (1992)	India	Chandigarh (urban)	First contacts, 1978–80	All help agencies	CATEGO S + CATEGO S,P,O or clinical diagnosis
Jablensky et al. (1992)	Ireland	Dublin	First contacts, 1978–80	All help agencies	CATEGO S + CATEGO S,P,O or clinical diagnosis
Jablensky et al. (1992)	USA	Honolulu, Hawaii	First contacts, 1978–80	All help agencies	CATEGO S + CATEGO S,P,O or clinical diagnosis
Jablensky et al. (1992)	USSR	Moscow	First contacts, 1978–81	All help agencies	CATEGO S + CATEGO S,P,O or clinical diagnosis
Jablensky et al. (1992)	Japan	Nagasaki	First contacts, 1978–80	All help agencies	CATEGO S + CATEGO S,P,O or clinical diagnosis
Jablensky et al. (1992)	UK	Nottingham	First contacts, 1978–80	All help agencies	CATEGO S + CATEGO S,P,O or clinical diagnosis
Tien & Eaton (1992)	USA	New Haven, CT	Representative sample of general population	Census survey, two waves	DIS/DSM-III, non-clinician interviewers

	Incidence per 1000 population per year					
Age group for calcu-lation of rate (years)	Narrow diagnosis		Standard diagnosis		Broad diagnosis	
	Without age correction	With age correction	Without age correction	With age correction	Without age correction	With age correction
15–54		0.11		0.42		
15–54		0.09		0.35		
15–54		0.09		0.22		
15–54		0.09		0.16		
15–54		0.12		0.28		
15–54		0.10		0.21		
15–54		0.14		0.24		
> 18				1.00		

Table 2 (cont.)

Authors	Country or area	Population	Sample	Case-finding method	Diagnostic assessment
Tien & Eaton (1992)	USA	Baltimore, MD	Representative sample of general population	Census survey, two waves	DIS/DSM-III, non-clinician interviewers
Tien & Eaton (1992)	USA	St Louis, MO	Representative sample of general population	Census survey, two waves	DIS/DSM-III, non-clinician interviewers
Tien & Eaton (1992)	USA	Durham, NC	Representative sample of general population	Census survey, two waves	DIS/DSM-III, non-clinician interviewers
Tien & Eaton (1992)	USA	Los Angeles, CA	Representative sample of general population	Census survey, two waves	DIS/DSM-III, non-clinician interviewers

a DIS interviewer skipped over a series of questions relating to schizophrenia because the subject responded to the first question in the section in a threatening manner. Patients who were coded as schizophrenic by the DIS were often diagnosed as suffering from some other mental disorder, such as bipolar disorder or histrionic personality, by the clinical interview.

The central problem in interpreting the unusual results from the ECA study is the extent to which the findings are the result of biases produced by the use of lay interviewers and a symptom questionnaire instead of face-to-face psychiatric evaluation.

3.1.2 The WHO Study on the Determinants of the Outcome of Severe Mental Disorders

The clearest indication of limited variability in the incidence of schizophrenia is the evidence from the WHO ten-country study of the incidence and course of

	Incidence per 1000 population per year					
Age group for calcu-lation of rate (years)	Narrow diagnosis		Standard diagnosis		Broad diagnosis	
	Without age correction	With age correction	Without age correction	With age correction	Without age correction	With age correction
> 18				7.10		
> 18				1.00		
> 18				1.60		
> 18				1.70		

schizophrenia (Jablensky et al., 1992). This multicentre study applied stand-ardized diagnostic criteria and used a thorough case-finding procedure which attempted to ensure that all people suffering from the disorder were included. The study set out to identify all those aged 15–54 who had either experienced a psychotic symptom or demonstrated psychotic behaviour during the previous year and who had made contact with a "helping agency" for psychiatric reasons for the first time in their lives. The help-givers included psychiatric and medical facilities, traditional healers, priests and other religious figures.

The study detected very little variation in the incidence of the illness between sites (see Fig. 1). The range for the most restrictive diagnostic category (CATEGO S +) was from 0.07 per 1000 in Aarhus, Denmark, to 0.14 in Nottingham, United Kingdom (mean 0.10 per 1000; SD 0.02). The broader diagnostic approach (a clinical diagnosis of schizophrenia or CATEGO S,P,O) produced a range of incidence values from 0.16 per 1000 in Honolulu, Hawaii, to 0.42 per 1000 in a rural area near Chandigarh, India: the mean was 0.25 per 1000 (SD = 0.09).

Fig. 1

Annual incidence of schizophrenia per 100 000 population aged 15 54 (both sexes) for the broad and restrictive definitions

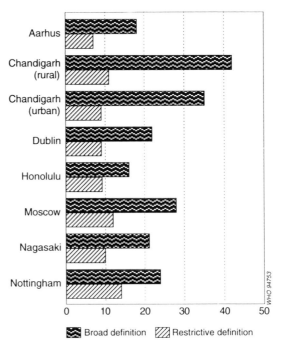

Broad definition   Restrictive definition

3.1.3 Incidence in developing countries

The symptom profiles of schizophrenic subjects in developed and developing countries are similar, with the following exceptions. Affective symptoms, especially depression, are more common among patients in developed countries. Some Schneiderian first-rank symptoms, such as thought insertion and thought broadcasting, occur more frequently in patients in developed countries while others, such as delusions of control, are more common in patients in developing countries. Auditory hallucinations and, particularly, visual hallucinations are more prevalent in the developing world. The two groups of patients are equally likely to experience the various kinds of delusions.

Torrey (1980) has argued, using prevalence data, that schizophrenia occurs less frequently in the developing world than in the developed world. The WHO ten-country study is of particular interest, therefore, in furnishing data on the incidence of schizophrenia in the Third World. These data reveal that the incidence of schizophrenia in Chandigarh, India, and in the rural area around the city is very similar to rates found in the developed world, when the restrictive CATEGO S + diagnostic standard is applied. Using a broader diagnostic approach, the rates in and around Chandigarh are above the mean for the centres in the developed world. Another study gave an incidence figure for the Haidan district of China of 0.11 per 1000 (Shen Yucun et al., 1981) which is below the mean for developed countries, but well within one standard deviation. A study from Madras, India (Rajkumar et al., 1991), detected a relatively high age-corrected incidence rate of 0.58 per 1000. Given the similarity in incidence figures for developed and developing countries, we must conclude that the low prevalence estimates for schizophrenia in the Third World (see section 3.2) are a consequence of higher recovery rates in the developing countries, which have been well documented (WHO, 1979; Warner, 1983; Jablensky et al., 1992), and, perhaps, of higher death rates among people suffering from psychosis.

3.1.4 Pockets of high incidence

Pockets of high levels of occurrence of schizophrenia have been reported in different parts of the world. Some of these reports, for example from the Istrian peninsula of Yugoslavia (Crocetti et al., 1971) and from a district of Sweden inside the Arctic Circle (Böök, 1953; Böök et al., 1978), rely upon prevalence estimates and may, therefore, be influenced by migration, recovery and death rates.

Unusually high incidence figures have been reported, none the less, for parts of Ireland. First admission rates for schizophrenia to Irish hospitals have been reported to be 2–3 times greater than those to hospitals in England and Wales (Walsh & Walsh, 1970). A recent report (Ní Nualláin et al., 1987), however, suggests that these "first admission" rates are somewhat exaggerated because many Irish hospitals interpreted "first admission" as first admission to *that* hospital, even though the patient may have been previously admitted elsewhere. A more rigorous investigation using standardized case-finding procedures and diagnostic guidelines (Ní Nualláin et al., 1987) has determined the incidence rate in three Irish counties with diverse characteristics to be above the mean, but not dramatically so. In this study, the age-corrected incidence of "core" schizophrenia (CATEGO S +) was 0.17 per 1000, compared with a mean of 0.11 for studies worldwide. The rate for a standard definition of schizophrenia (ICD 295, 297) was 0.37, which is within one standard deviation of the worldwide mean of 0.26. In the WHO ten-country study the incidence of schizophrenia in Dublin (CATEGO S + , 0.12; standard diagnosis, 0.24) was very close to the worldwide mean. A recent review of epidemiological studies suggests that Ireland should not be considered to have a high incidence of schizophrenia without more reliable research (Cabot, 1990). In Ireland, as elsewhere, the apparent variability in the frequency of occurrence of schizophrenia diminishes as the research methodology becomes more standardized.

High incidence figures have also been reported for parts of Germany. Häfner & Reimann (1970) reported a rate of 0.54 per 1000 (not age-corrected) in Mannheim, and Häfner & Gattaz (1991) reported a rate of 0.56 per 1000 for the same city at a later date. Dilling & Weyerer (1980) similarly reported a rate of 0.48 per 1000 in upper Bavaria. Each of these studies based the incidence rate upon a case register and the diagnosis of the treating facility, which may have been unusually broad. This explanation is supported by the finding of Häfner & Gattaz (1991) that the incidence of narrowly defined (CATEGO S +) schizophrenia in the same region of Germany, at 0.09 per 1000, was not above the worldwide mean.

Somewhat elevated incidence figures have also been reported for India. Rajkumar et al. (1991) found an age-corrected rate of 0.58 per 1000 in Madras and, as mentioned above, higher than average rates were found in the WHO study in Chandigarh city and in the surrounding rural area (0.35 and 0.42 per 1000, age-corrected). The incidence rate found using the narrow definition (CATEGO S +), however, was not elevated in and around Chandigarh.

3.1.5 Differences in age of onset for males and females

A common finding of incidence studies of schizophrenia, and one which was noted by Kraepelin in 1909, is that the onset of the disorder is earlier in males than in females. Earlier onset of schizophrenia in men, as assessed on the basis of the first hospitalization, was found in five out of seven centres included in the WHO Collaborative Study on Assessment and Reduction of Psychiatric Disability (Hambrecht et al., 1992). In a review of more than 50 studies, Angermayer & Kuhn (1988) found age differences ranging from one to ten years between men and women at first admission. The difference is apparent regardless of the definition of onset used: whether the date of first hospital admission (the measure used by Kraepelin), for example, the occurrence of the first symptoms of schizophrenia, or the occurrence of the first nonspecific signs of a mental disorder or personality change.

A study conducted through the Danish National Psychiatric Case Register and the Mannheim case register yielded useful information on sex differences in age at first admission. Hospital admissions for schizophrenia and related diagnoses and previous admissions for other diagnoses were compared for cohorts of the Danish population and of inhabitants of Mannheim for specific years (Häfner et al., 1989). The authors found that first admission to hospital was 5–6 years earlier in men than in women in both countries when broad diagnostic criteria were employed, and 4–5 years earlier when a restrictive definition was applied. The finding was not attributable to diagnostic procedures or to sex differences in seeking help or occupational status. There was no difference in age at first hospitalization, however, between single men and women. This observation could indicate either a protective effect of marriage on women's vulnerability to schizophrenia or a reduction in marriage rates in women who have an earlier onset of the disorder. Riecher-Rössler et al. (1992), re-analysing the German data, concluded that there was no evidence to support the first hypothesis.

In a two-year study in Germany Häfner et al. (1992) found that the earliest signs of mental disturbance occurred four and a half years prior to first

Table 3
Mean age at different points in the development of schizophrenia for men and women, Germany

	Age (years)	
	Men	Women
Earliest sign of mental disturbance	24.3	27.5
First schizophrenic symptom	26.5	30.6
Beginning of "Index" episode	27.8	31.7
Admission for "Index" episode	28.5	32.4

admission, on average. The onset was significantly earlier in males than females regardless of the operational definition of onset used. Table 3 shows the mean age at different points in the development of the disorder for men and women. Recently Faraone et al. (1994) demonstrated that the observed earlier onset of illness in males is not due to demographic confounding.

In Häfner's sample, schizophrenia started with negative symptoms in 70% of the cases, the earliest negative symptom appearing on average six years before the first admission. Positive symptoms followed, appearing no earlier than two years before the first admission. Core symptomatology at the beginning of the psychosis and the progress of positive and negative symptoms were similar in both sexes and all age groups studied.

Women have a lower rate of development of schizophrenia than males in adolescence, but show a second peak in incidence after the menopause. Häfner (1991) argued that this pattern suggests a connection between the onset of the disorder and estrogen secretion: estradiol may produce a neuroleptic-like effect on dopamine secretion and on prolactin levels and thus may reduce the vulnerability to schizophrenia. This hypothesis has been confirmed to some extent by experimental studies (Häfner et al., 1991a, 1991b). The sex difference in the age of onset, moreover, appears to be true in different countries, an observation that supports a biological explanation, rather than a psychosocial one.

The overall incidence of schizophrenia in men and women is similar in most studies. Häfner (1991) found that the cumulative incidence up to age 60, an indicator of the lifetime risk, was equal for females and males. This suggests that whatever factors account for the sex differences in the disorder only serve to delay the onset and do not prevent it. A few studies, nevertheless, have found a significantly higher incidence of schizophrenia among males than among females (Iacono & Beiser, 1992). In the WHO DOSMED study, when paranoid and selected reactive states were excluded from the schizophrenia spectrum, six of the eight sites reported an excess of males over females (Jablensky et al., 1992). It is possible that gender bias may explain the under-representation of women found in some studies (Hambrecht et al., 1992). In a recent study designed to overcome previous methodological problems, no significant differences in the incidence of schizophrenia in men and women could be detected using a variety of diagnostic definitions (Hambrecht et al., 1994).

The later onset in women may partially explain the observation that the illness is less severe in women than in men. As early as 1845, the British physician, John Thurnam (1845), noted that the proportion of asylum patients discharged as recovered was consistently higher for females than males. A century later, Ödegaard (1960) found a higher early discharge rate for females than males among schizophrenics leaving Norwegian hospitals between 1936 and 1945. Beck (1978) noted that outcome studies often demonstrate a worse outcome for male schizophrenics, and never for females. In the WHO International Pilot Study of Schizophrenia, fewer women patients than men were in the worst outcome group at follow-up and more women than men were in the best outcome group.

The superior outcome for female schizophrenic patients may be due to biological factors, such as the anti-dopaminergic effect of estrogen, decreased cerebral laterality in women or lower rates of perinatal complications in female infants (Seeman, 1982); social factors, such as reduced labour market stress (Warner, 1985); or simply the later onset of illness in women (Lewine, 1981). Later onset provides an opportunity for the development of a higher level of premorbid social competence and is a predictor of good outcome in schizophrenia (Phillips, 1953; Stephens et al., 1966; Marder et al., 1979). Data from four psychiatric case registers in Australia, Denmark, the United Kingdom and the United States of America (Eaton et al., 1992b) suggest that sex differences in the course of schizophrenia are explained by the earlier age of onset in men. In each of the four areas, early age of onset was associated with an increased risk of readmission to hospital. When age of onset was taken into account, neither sex nor marital status had significant effects on risk of rehospitalization.

3.2 Prevalence studies

3.2.1 Community studies

Studies of the prevalence of schizophrenia in the general population give an impression of considerable variation. The same methodological problems that contribute to the apparent variation in incidence statistics apply to prevalence studies, and are amplified by differences in recovery rates, migration and death rates. An additional source of variation is the period of time over which prevalence is estimated. The number of cases at any one time is the *point prevalence*; the number observed in a given period (often one year) is the *period prevalence*; and the number in the population who have suffered from the illness at any time in their lives is the *lifetime prevalence*. Lifetime prevalence is unaffected by recovery rates but is influenced by the rate of migration and death among affected persons.

The studies listed in Table 4 display a wide variation in prevalence rates, even among those using roughly similar epidemiological approaches. In studies measuring point prevalence or prevalence for a period of up to one year,

Table 4
Studies of the prevalence of schizophrenia

Authors	Country or area	Population	Type of study[a]	Age group surveyed (years)	Period	Prevalence per 1000 population	
						without age correction	with age correction
Europe							
Temkov et al. (1980)	Bulgaria	urban	s.c.	–	point	2.8	
Folnegović & Folnegović-Šmalc (1992)	Croatia	urban or rural	census	20–64	3 months		5.1
Folnegović & Folnegović-Šmalc (1992)	Croatia	urban or rural	census	20–64	3 months		3.5
Folnegović & Folnegović-Šmalc (1992)	Croatia	urban or rural	census	20–64	3 months		1.5
Strömgren (1938)	Denmark	rural & small town	census	–	lifetime	3.3	
Fremming (1951)	Denmark	rural & small town	b.c.	51–56	lifetime		8.2
Nielsen & Nielsen (1977)	Denmark	rural	census	> 14	lifetime	2.2	2.7
Kaila (1942)	Finland	rural	census	–	lifetime	4.3	
Väisänen (1975)	Finland	rural	census	15–64	point	15.0	15.1
Lehtinen et al. (1978)	Finland	rural	census	–	point		1.3
Lehtinen et al. (1990a)	Finland	urban & rural	census	18–64	point		2.7
Lehtinen et al. (1990b)	Finland	urban & rural	b.c.	30–80	point		2.4
Brugger (1931)	Germany	rural	census	> 10	lifetime	1.9	
Brugger (1933)	Germany	rural	census	–	lifetime	2.2	
Klemperer (1933)	Germany		b.c.	–	point	10.0	
Brugger (1938)	Germany	rural	census	> 10	lifetime	1.8	2.3
Dilling & Weyerer (1984)	Germany, Fed. Rep. of	rural	census	> 15	point		3.9
Helgason (1964)	Iceland	urban & rural	b.c.	60–62	lifetime		6.0
Stefánsson et al. (1991)	Iceland	urban & rural	census	55–57	lifetime		0.4
Walsh (1976)	Ireland	rural	s.c.	> 15	point		7.6
Walsh et al. (1980)	Ireland	rural	s.c.	> 14	point	7.1	9.8
Torrey et al. (1984)	Ireland	rural	census	> 14	6 months	12.6	17.4
Youssef et al. (1991)	Ireland	rural	census	> 14	1 year	3.3	4.6

37

Table 4 (cont.)

Authors	Country or area	Population	Type of study[a]	Age group surveyed (years)	Period	Prevalence per 1000 population	
						without age correction	with age correction
Zimmerman-Tansella et al. (1985)	Italy	urban	s.c.	>13	1 year		1.3
Bremer (1951)	Norway	rural	census	>9	lifetime	4.5	5.6
Fugelli (1975)	Norway	rural	census	>19	2 years	5.8	8.9
Vazquez-Barquero et al. (1987)	Spain	rural	census	>17	point		5.6
Sjögren (1948), Larsson & Sjögren (1954)	Sweden	rural	census	>15	45 years	5.6	7.2
Böök (1953)	Sweden	rural	census	>14	48 years	9.5	15.8
Essen-Moller (1956)	Sweden	rural	census	>15	lifetime	6.7	9.4
Hagnell (1966)	Sweden	rural	census	>10	lifetime	4.5	5.1
Böök et al. (1978)	Sweden	rural	census	–	77 years	17.0	
Halldin (1984)	Sweden	urban	census	18–65	1 year		6.0
Widerlov et al. (1989)	Sweden	urban	s.c.	18–64	lifetime		5.0
Widerlov et al. (1989)	Sweden	rural	s.c.	18–64	lifetime		0.7
Mayer-Gross (1948)	UK (Scotland)	rural	census	–	lifetime	4.2	
Primrose (1962)	UK (Scotland)	rural	census	>14	point	1.8	2.4
Wing et al. (1967)	UK	urban	s.c.	>14	1 year	3.4	4.4
Wing & Fryers (1976)	UK	urban	s.c.	–	point	1.8	
Freeman & Alpert (1986)	UK	urban	s.c.	>14	1 year		6.8
Mavreas & Bebbington (1987)	UK	urban	census	>18	point		13.0
Bamrah et al. (1991)	UK	urban	s.c.	>14	1 year		7.5
Zharikov (1968)	USSR	urban	s.c.	>15	point	3.6	5.1
Rotstein (1977)	USSR	several areas	census	–	point	3.8	
Ouspenskaya (1978)	USSR	various areas	s.c.	>13	lifetime		5.3
Crocetti et al. (1971)	Yugoslavia	urban	census	20–64	3 months		7.3
Crocetti et al. (1971)	Yugoslavia	urban	census	20–64	3 months		4.2
Kulcar et al. (1971)	Yugoslavia	rural	census	20–64	3 months		7.4

North America

Study	Country	Setting	Sampling	Age	Prevalence	Rate	Rate
Leighton et al. (1963)	Canada	rural	census	>17	point		5.0
Murphy & Lemieux (1967)	Canada	"old French" villages	census	>14	point		10.5
Murphy & Lemieux (1967)	Canada	"new French" villages	census	>14	point		7.1
Murphy & Lemieux (1967)	Canada	"Anglo-Protestant" villages	census	>14	point		4.2
Murphy & Lemieux (1967)	Canada	"Irish-Catholic" villages	census	>14	point		7.1
Murphy & Lemieux (1967)	Canada	"Polish" villages	census	>14	point		7.2
Murphy & Lemieux (1967)	Canada	"German" villages	census	>14	point		5.8
Bland et al. (1988)	Canada	urban	census	>18	lifetime		0.3
Lemkau et al. (1942, 1943)	USA	urban	census	—	lifetime	2.9	
Roth & Luton (1943)	USA	rural	census	—	lifetime	2.0	
Hollingshead & Redlich (1958)	USA	urban	census	—	6 months	3.6	
Kramer (1978)	USA	urban	census	>14	1 year	4.7	6.4
Weissman & Myers (1980)	USA	urban	census	>18	point		4.0
Myers et al. (1984)	USA	urban	census	>17	6 months		6.0
Myers et al. (1984)	USA	urban	census	>17	6 months		10.0
Myers et al. (1984)	USA	urban	census	>17	6 months		11.0
Blazer et al. (1985)	USA	rural	census	>17	6 months		6.0
Blazer et al. (1985)	USA	rural	census	>17	6 months		11.0
Burnam et al. (1987)	USA	urban	census	>18	6 months		3.0
Burnam et al. (1987)	USA	urban	census	>18	6 months		6.0
Canino et al. (1987)	Puerto Rico	urban and rural	census	18–64	6 months		15.0
Babigian (1980)	USA	urban	s.c.	—	1 year	4.1	

Japan

Study	Country	Setting	Sampling	Age	Prevalence	Rate	Rate
Uchimura (1940)	Japan	rural	census	—	lifetime		3.8
Mukasa et al. (1941)	Japan	rural	census	—	lifetime		3.2
Hiratsuka & Nomura (1941)	Japan	rural	census	—	lifetime		4.1
Tsugawa (1942)	Japan	urban	census	—	lifetime		2.2
Akimoto et al. (1943)	Japan	small town	census	—	lifetime		2.1
Ogino & Nagao (1943)	Japan	rural	census	—	lifetime		2.4

Table 4 (cont.)

Authors	Country or area	Population	Type of study[a]	Age group surveyed (years)	Period	Prevalence per 1000 population	
						without age correction	with age correction
Japanese Ministry of Health & Welfare (1955)	Japan	urban & rural	census	–	1 year	2.3	
Okabe (1957)	Japan	rural	census	–	lifetime	7.4	
Arai et al. (1958)	Japan	rural	census	–	lifetime	11.2	
Arai et al. (1958)	Japan	rural	census	–	lifetime	2.8	
Arai et al. (1958)	Japan	rural	census	–	lifetime	5.0	
Akimoto et al. (1964)	Japan	rural	census	–	lifetime	4.7	
Japanese Ministry of Health & Welfare (1965)	Japan	urban & rural	census	–	1 year	2.3	
Sato (1966)	Japan	urban	census	–	5 years	2.8	
Hirayasu (1969)	Japan	rural	census	–	lifetime	8.8	
Kato (1969)	Japan	rural	census	–	lifetime	4.7	
Haruki (1972)	Japan	rural	census	–	lifetime	8.5	
Shibata et al. (1975)	Japan	rural	census	–	lifetime	1.9	
Shibata et al. (1978)	Japan	rural	census	–	lifetime	17.9	
Special populations in developed countries							
Jones & Horne (1973)	Australia (western)	Aborigines	census	>16	point	4.7	9.3
Eastwell (1975)	Australia (northern)	Aborigines	census	>16	point	5.0	9.9
Roy et al. (1970)	Canada	Indians	census	>14	point	5.7	11.0
Roy et al. (1970)	Canada	non-Indians	census	>14	point	1.6	2.4
Eaton & Weil (1955)	Canada	Hutterites	census	>14	lifetime	1.1	2.1
Egeland & Hostetter (1983)	USA	Amish	census	>14	5 years	0.3	0.5
Developing countries							
Ben-Tovim & Cushnie (1986)	Botswana	rural	census	>14	1 year		5.3
Lin et al. (1981)	China	rural & urban	census	–	point	4.2	
Shen Yucun et al. (1981)	China	rural & urban	s.c.	–	point	1.8	
Cheung (1991)	China	rural	census	–	1 year	1.9	

Study	Country	Setting	Method	Age	Period		
Cheung (1991)	China	rural	census	—	1 year	2.6	
Cheung (1991)	China	12 regions	census	—	1 year	4.7	
Cheung (1991)	China	12 regions	census	—	lifetime	5.7	
Cheung (1991)	China	rural	census	—	1 year	2.2	
Lin (1953)	China (Province of Taiwan)	Chinese	census	>10	lifetime	2.2	3.1
Rin & Lin (1962)	China (Province of Taiwan)	Aborigines	census	—	lifetime	0.9	
Lin et al. (1969)	China (Province of Taiwan)	Chinese	census	>10	lifetime	1.4	2.0
Hwu et al. (1989)	China (Province of Taiwan)	Chinese	census	>18	lifetime		2.5
Sikanerty & Eaton (1984)	Ghana	rural	census	>14	point	0.6	1.1
Surya et al. (1964)	India	urban	census	>14	point	1.5	2.6
Sethi et al. (1967)	India	urban	census	>10	point	2.3	3.4
Elnagar et al. (1971)	India	rural	census	>14	point	4.3	8.0
Dube & Kumar (1972)	India	urban & rural	census	>14	lifetime	2.2	3.7
Sethi et al. (1972a)	India	urban	census	—	point	2.4	
Sethi et al. (1972b)	India	rural	census	>10	point	1.1	1.7
Verghese et al. (1973)	India	urban	census	>12	point	1.7	2.6
Sethi et al. (1974)	India	urban	census	>10	point	2.5	2.9
Nandi et al. (1975)	India	rural	census	—	point	2.8	
Thacore et al. (1975)	India	urban	census	>15	point	1.9	3.3
Carstairs & Kapur (1976)	India	rural	census	>14	point		7.2
Murthy et al. (1978)	India	rural	census	—	point	7.0	
Nandi et al. (1980)	India	rural	census	—	point	2.2	
Lee et al. (1990a)	Republic of Korea	rural	census	>18	lifetime		5.4
Lee et al. (1990b)	Republic of Korea	urban	census	>18	lifetime		3.1
Jayasundera (1969)	Sri Lanka	semi-rural	census	—	point	3.2	
Jayasundera (1969)	Sri Lanka	semi-rural	census	—	point	2.3	
Jayasundera (1969)	Sri Lanka	rural	census	—	point	5.2	
Jayasundera (1969)	Sri Lanka	traditional rural	census	—	point	1.3	
Wijesinghe et al. (1978)	Sri Lanka	semi-urban	census	>14	6 months	3.7	5.5
Baasher (1961)	Sudan	village	census	—	point	7.0	
Murphy & Taumoepeau (1980)	Tonga	rural	census	>10	1 year	0.4	0.9
Murphy & Taumoepeau (1980)	Tonga	rural	census	>10	1 year	0.7	1.3

[a] b,c = birth cohort study; census = census (including key informant) study; s.c. = service contact study.

age-corrected rates range from a low of 0.9 per 1000 of the population in Tonga to a high of 17.4 per 1000 in Ireland, with a mean of 5.8 per 1000 (SD 3.6).

This variation in prevalence has been remarked upon in a number of recent reviews (Eaton, 1985; Eaton et al., 1988; Torrey, 1987). Torrey (1987) argued that the data supported the possibility of a real tenfold difference in prevalence, comparable to the prevalence range reported for rheumatoid arthritis. He also pointed out that the north–south gradient in the distribution of schizophrenia is similar to that reported for heart disease and multiple sclerosis.

A more restricted prevalence range was noted by Jablensky (1986) in his review of 26 European epidemiological studies carried out among geographically defined populations: he found a point prevalence in the range 2.5–5.3 per 1000, and an individual morbidity risk between 0.36% and 1.87%.

As Jablensky (1988) pointed out, there is another syndrome with a heterogeneous etiology and a similar pattern of distribution over geographical areas and time, namely mental retardation. Häfner (1988) argued, similarly, that vulnerability to schizophrenia may be distributed along a continuous dimension in the population, as are low IQ values. Different disorders in the schizophrenia spectrum, he suggested, are arranged along this dimension from severe psychosis, through intermediate disorders, to mental health. A restrictive definition of schizophrenia, such as CATEGO S + , will capture a certain proportion of the cases, just as a low cut-off score for IQ will capture a small proportion of those considered mentally retarded. Broader diagnostic criteria will capture a larger section of the people with disorders in the schizophrenia spectrum.

3.2.2 Prevalence in developing countries

Prevalence figures for developing-country populations are consistently lower than those in the developed world. For example, a number of surveys carried out on large samples in China between 1980 and 1985, using a two-stage procedure and, in some instances, employing the PSE for the second stage assessment, found low period prevalence rates ranging between 1.9 per 1000 and 4.7 per 1000 (Cheung, 1991).

Age-corrected point or one-year prevalence rates in the studies in Table 4 from developing countries average 3.4 per 1000 (range 0.9 to 8.0; SD 2.09) compared with a mean rate of 6.3 per 1000 (range 1.3 to 17.4; SD 4.32) in Europe and North America. The difference between these means is significant at the 0.001 level (Student's *t* test). Given the similarity in incidence rates in the developed and developing worlds, the difference in prevalence rates is unlikely to be due to a disparity in the rate of occurrence of schizophrenia. It is more likely to be the result of difficulties in locating cases, higher death rates and (in the case of point and period prevalence rates) higher recovery rates from schizophrenia in developing countries.

One report indicated high prevalence rates for psychosis in one area of the developing world. In a recent review of epidemiological research conducted in seven countries of Central and South America, a median prevalence rate for functional psychoses of 11 per 1000 was determined, with a range between 2 and 86 per 1000 (Levav et al., 1989). This unusually high median prevalence figure and the wide range of rates are likely to be the result of variations between the studies in diagnostic and case-finding methods, including the use of the DIS which, as explained above, yields inappropriately high occurrence rates for schizophrenia.

3.2.3 Pockets of high and low prevalence

Pockets of increased prevalence of schizophrenia have been found in different parts of the world, including arctic districts of Sweden (77-year prevalence of 17.0 per 1000) (Böök et al., 1978), arctic Finland (age-corrected point prevalence of 15.1 per 1000) (Väisänen, 1975) and the west of Ireland (age-corrected six-month prevalence of 17.4 per 1000) (Torrey et al., 1984). Each of these areas is characterized by high levels of emigration associated with harsh subsistence conditions and land shortage. The same is true for the Istrian peninsula, which has been shown to have a higher prevalence of schizophrenia than the remainder of Croatia (Crocetti et al., 1971). It is probable that these prevalence figures are artificially elevated by both the out-migration of healthy individuals and the return to their original homes of people who fall ill abroad. In one prevalence study of schizophrenia in the west of Ireland (Torrey et al., 1984), for example, 14% of the patients reported that most or all of their siblings had emigrated, making it likely that the person's illness had precluded emigration, and a further 19% of the patients had themselves emigrated and returned for reasons probably or possibly connected with their illness. Thus, a third of the reported prevalence rate in the region could be accounted for by the effect of migration. In the west of Ireland, furthermore, accurate, standardized incidence data have recently been gathered, and no elevation in the occurrence of schizophrenia was detected (Ní Nualláin et al., 1987).

Migration and other non-etiological factors, therefore, probably account for the observed high prevalence rates in Ireland and other areas. Other explanations may also apply: in arctic Sweden, for example, the population is a genetic isolate and the high prevalence of schizophrenia has been traced to a genetic founder effect.

Migration appears to be one of the most significant factors determining prevalence rates in Croatia. A recent study conducted there (Folnegović & Folnegović-Šmalc, 1992) revealed that the prevalence of schizophrenia and the risk of admission to hospital were greatest in the district where emigration rates were highest, and lowest in the districts where immigration rates were highest. There was little variation between districts, however, in first-admission rates, which are an indicator of incidence. This finding suggests that the effect of migration is restricted to the current generation of cases and is not cumulative over time.

Migration effects may also help account for the unusually high and low prevalence rates for schizophrenia found in certain segregated populations in the developed world. Two conservative Anabaptist agrarian sects in North America, for example, have been shown to have unusually low prevalence rates of schizophrenia and high rates of affective disorder. The Hutterite Brethren of the north-western United States of America and western Canada have been shown by Eaton & Weil (1955) to have an age-corrected lifetime prevalence of schizophrenia as low as 2.1 per 1000. Similarly, the Old Order Amish, who live in farming communities across North America, have a very low age-corrected five-year prevalence for schizophrenia of 0.5 per 1000 (Egeland & Hostetter, 1983). This pattern of occurrence could be explained by a lack of tolerance for deviant behaviour in these conservative communities and the out-migration of psychotic and pre-psychotic individuals. The high prevalence in these communities of affective disorder, including bipolar illness, however, argues against this explanation. Alternative interpretations of the data include a diagnostic bias in both studies favouring bipolar disorder over schizophrenia, a sociocultural effect on the true occurrence of these disorders (Warner, 1985) or a limited genetic vulnerability to schizophrenia among the founder members of both sects.

A high prevalence of schizophrenia has been found in some discrete populations living on the margin of the industrial world. An elevated age-corrected point prevalence of schizophrenia of 11.0 per 1000, for example, has been identified among the Cree and Salteaux Indians of northern Saskatchewan, Canada. This is in marked contrast to the low rate of 2.4 per 1000 for non-Indians living in the same region (Roy et al., 1970). High rates of unemployment and dependence characterize the Indian population in this region, whereas the local white population enjoys a more stable agrarian economy. Out-migration of healthy individuals from the Indian community may explain the high rate of schizophrenia. A similar phenomenon may explain the relatively high prevalence rates of schizophrenia among Aboriginals living in dependent communities around government-sustained missions in various parts of Australia (Jones & Horne, 1973; Eastwell, 1975). Disabled members of the Aboriginal population may be more likely to remain in these communities while healthier members migrate to areas with better employment opportunities. A social effect on the occurrence of the disorder, however, cannot be excluded. It is possible that the risk of schizophrenia is increased in populations where exposure to western lifestyles disturbs pre-existing cultural isolation (Jablensky & Sartorius, 1975; Warner, 1985).

3.2.4 The Epidemiologic Catchment Area study

The large-scale ECA survey has provided a good deal of information about the epidemiology and the sociodemographic and clinical features of schizophrenia (Keith et al., 1991). As described in section 3.1.1, however, the incidence of schizophrenia detected in this study was substantially greater than that identified in other research—a finding that appears to be a result of the use of non-clinician interviewers producing an unusually high number of false-positive results. In the ECA study, the lifetime prevalence of schizophrenia, according to DIS/DSM-III criteria, was determined to be 14 per 1000 of the population, substantially above the mean of 5.5 per 1000 for lifetime prevalence for the studies conducted in North America and Europe listed in Table 4. It is probable that many of the cases identified by the DIS were not, in fact, schizophrenia; for this reason further data on demographic and clinical features of these cases are not presented here.

A recent study in the USA, the National Comorbidity Survey, has confirmed the impression that the prevalence of schizophrenia in the ECA study was elevated by artefacts. The National Comorbidity Survey used lay interviewers to administer a revised version of the CIDI to a national probability sample of 8098 people. The authors found lifetime and 12-month prevalence rates of "nonaffective psychosis" (schizophrenia, schizophreniform disorder, schizoaffective disorder, delusional disorder, and atypical psychosis, diagnosed according to the DSM-III-R criteria) to be respectively 7 and 5 per 1000 population aged 15–54 years. This lifetime rate is substantially lower than the ECA figure.

3.2.5 Family and twin studies

It has been observed that some of the most striking advances in research on schizophrenia in the past 25 years have been in the field of genetics (Eaton, 1985). Family studies have made a valuable contribution to understanding the origins of schizophrenia.

In family studies that include people of widely differing ages, it is useful to calculate the lifetime *morbid risk*—the likelihood that someone will suffer an episode of illness between birth and death—rather than the actual rate of development of the illness. The Weinberg method of calculating morbid risk, which adjusts observed occurrence rates to allow for the age of the subjects is commonly used.

If genetic factors are important in the development of schizophrenia, one would expect that morbid risk would be higher in relatives of people with the illness than in the general population, and that the risk would be greater in those with a closer genetic relationship. Gottesman (1991), drawing data from about 40 European studies conducted between 1920 and 1987, calculated the average morbid risk of developing schizophrenia for people with different degrees of relationship to someone with schizophrenia. The results, displayed in Fig. 2, indicate that the risk varies with the extent of gene-sharing. Thus the risk is greatest in the identical twins of schizophrenics (48% risk) and decreases step by step in the children of two schizophrenic parents, first-degree relatives, second-degree relatives, third-degree relatives, and finally the general population (1% risk).

Fig. 2
Average risk of developing schizophrenia, according to relationship to a schizophrenic patient

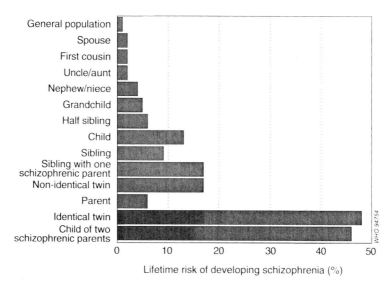

Lifetime risk of developing schizophrenia (%)

From Gottesman (1991).

The observed data suggest that genetic factors are important in the development of schizophrenia but are not sufficient to explain completely the pattern of occurrence. Monozygotic twins, although genetically identical, are concordant for schizophrenia in only about half of the cases; 89% of schizophrenic subjects do not have a schizophrenic parent, and 63% have no relative, of any degree of relatedness, with the illness (Gottesman, 1991).

Is the risk of schizophrenia elevated in the offspring of a schizophrenic individual because the child is raised by a mentally ill parent? Adoption studies provide information on this question. In Heston's (1966) Oregon study, the morbid risk of schizophrenia in the adopted offspring of schizophrenic mothers was 16.6% and, therefore, not lower than the average risk of 13% (Fig. 2) for offspring reared by their own schizophrenic parents. This finding suggests that exposure to a schizophrenic parent does not increase the risk of developing the illness.

A Danish adoption study using a different approach arrived at a similar conclusion. Kety and associates (Kety, 1988; Wender et al., 1974) evaluated the biological and adoptive parents of people in Copenhagen who had been adopted by non-relatives. As Table 5 shows, adopted offspring whose biological parents suffered from a disorder in the schizophrenia spectrum were nearly twice as likely as the offspring of non-schizophrenic parents to develop a schizophrenia-spectrum disorder themselves. The offspring of normal biological parents were equally likely to develop a schizophrenia-spectrum

Table 5

Schizophrenia-spectrum disorders in adopted children, according to presence of schizophrenia in biological and adoptive parents[a]

Parents		Adoptees with schizophrenia-spectrum disorders (%)
Biological	**Adoptive**	
Normal	Normal	10.7
Normal	Schizophrenia	10.7
Schizophrenia	Normal	18.8

[a]Adapted from Wender et al. (1974).

disorder whether they were raised by normal or schizophrenic adoptive parents (Wender et al., 1974). Again, the conclusion may be drawn that the risk of developing a schizophrenia-spectrum disorder is not increased by being raised by a parent with the same disorder.

Further evidence confirming the impression that the home environment does not contribute to the risk of developing schizophrenia is the finding that the concordance rate for the illness in identical twins is no lower in twins who are raised separately (64% concordance) than in those who are raised by their parents (48%) (Gottesman & Shields, 1982).

One adoptive study suggested that child-raising may have an effect on the development of schizophrenia. Tienari et al. (1987) examined children born in Finland between 1928 and 1979 to mothers afflicted with schizophrenia, and raised by adoptive parents, and compared them with a group of matched controls. As expected, schizophrenia appeared more frequently in the children of schizophrenic mothers. However, the adoptive families of the schizophrenic offspring were clinically rated as being more disturbed than the other families. The findings suggest that the appearance of schizophrenia may be the result of an interaction between genetic and environmental factors. It is probable, however, that the higher levels of disturbance in the adoptive families were, at least in part, a consequence of raising a severely disturbed schizophrenic or pre-schizophrenic child.

3.2.6 Season of birth

More than 40 articles have appeared on the season of birth of schizophrenic patients (Bradbury & Miller, 1985; Hare, 1988). The majority report an excess of births in late winter or spring among treated schizophrenics, the proportion born at this time being approximately 10% higher than at other times of the year (Eaton et al., 1988). The findings of the larger studies are illustrated in Fig. 3. Many possible reasons have been suggested for this finding, some artefactual and some etiological. They include:

Fig. 3
Months with higher-than-normal birth rate of schizophrenic subjects, selected studies[a]

Authors		No. of cases	Significance	Dec.	Jan.	Feb.	Mar.	Apr.	May	Jun.	Jul.	Aug.	Sep.	Oct.	Nov.
Northern hemisphere															
Tramer	1929	3 100	$P \leqslant 0.001$												
de Sauvage	1934/1951/1954	4 679	$P \leqslant 0.001$												
Hare & Price	1968	3 596	$P \leqslant 0.05$												
Dalén	1968	16 238	$P \leqslant 0.001$												
Hare et al.	1974	5 139	$P \leqslant 0.01$												
Ödegaard	1974	19 749	$P \leqslant 0.05$												
Videbech et al.	1974	7 427	$P \leqslant 0.001$												
Parker & Balza	1977	3 508	$P \leqslant 0.001$												
Shimura et al.	1977	5 431	$P \leqslant 0.01$												
Torrey et al.	1977	53 584	$P \leqslant 0.05$												
O'Hare et al.	1980	4 855	$P \leqslant 0.001$												
Watson et al.	1984	3 246	$P \leqslant 0.01$												
Kendell & Kemp	1985	3 224	$P \leqslant 0.05$												
Häfner et al.	1987	2 020	$P \leqslant 0.05$												
Southern hemisphere															
Dalén	1975	2 947	$P \leqslant 0.05$	(females only, $n = 1506$)											
Parker & Neilson	1976	2 256	$P \leqslant 0.01$	(females only, $n = 1195$)											

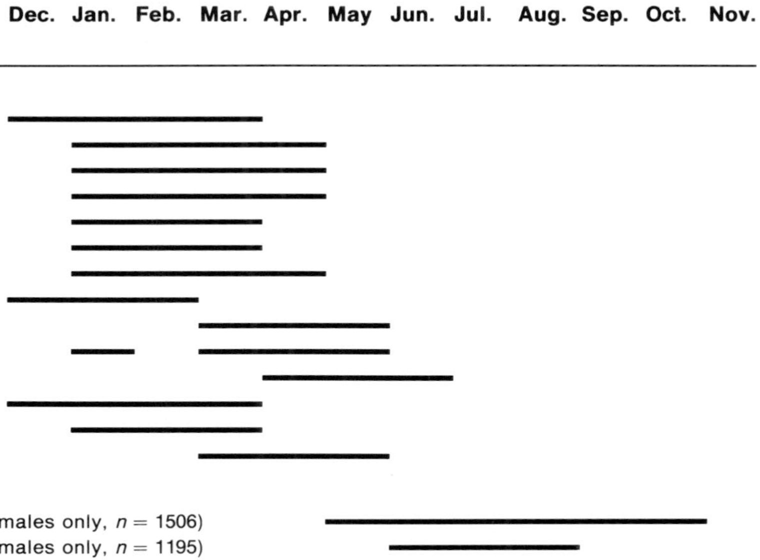

[a]Studies including fewer than 2000 cases are not listed.
From Häfner (1987)

(a) a statistical artefact referred to as an "age prevalence effect" (Lewis, 1989),
(b) a seasonal variation in the risk of premature delivery (Müller & Kleider, 1990),
(c) increased spring and summer mating of the parents of schizophrenics (Ödegaard, 1974),
(d) a seasonal effect on maternal endocrine and behavioural factors (Häfner, 1990),
(e) a higher proportion of older women giving birth early in the year (Dalén, 1990),
(f) nutritional effects, including haemorrhagic disease of newborn caused by vitamin K deficiency (Dalén, 1990),
(g) the effect on gestation of hot summers (Pasamanick, 1986), cool autumns (Kendell & Adams, 1991) or cold winters (Hare & Moran, 1981),
(h) the effect of influenza or other viral diseases during the second trimester of pregnancy (Watson et al., 1984; Mednick et al., 1987; Torrey et al., 1988; Barr et al., 1990),
(i) the effect of some other infectious agent with a seasonal periodicity similar to that of influenza (Torrey et al., 1988),
(j) the effect of drugs taken by the mother to combat the symptoms of influenza and other seasonal infections (Beiser & Iacono, 1990), and
(k) a genetic effect that increases the risk of schizophrenia but decreases the risk of perinatal death from winter infections (Pulver et al., 1992).

Lewis (1989) challenged the view that the excess of winter births in schizophrenia reflects an etiological effect and argued that it is the result of a distortion of the data caused by an artefact referred to as an "age prevalence" or "age incidence" effect. This statistical concept is based on the fact that older people have had more time to develop an illness such as schizophrenia than those who are younger. Within any year, therefore, people born in January or February are more likely to develop an illness than those born later in the year. This will be a relevant factor in any study that observes the usual convention of using the calendar year, beginning on January 1, to define the year of birth and the year of admission to hospital. In support of this view, Lewis pointed out several inconsistent findings in the literature, including a lack of consistency in establishing an excess of winter births in the southern hemisphere (where one would expect the age prevalence effect to be reversed). Some northern hemisphere studies, however, have applied the displacement test proposed by Lewis to correct for the age prevalence artefact (O'Callaghan et al., 1991), or have used a life table method to minimize the effect of the calendar year (Pulver et al., 1983), and have still observed a significant excess of winter births.

Eaton (1991) argued that the existence of an age prevalence or age incidence effect seems indisputable; it is unclear, however, whether the effect is sufficient to explain the birth pattern observed. He noted, "with only a 10% excess of schizophrenic births in the winter and spring, the age incidence effect will remain a strong candidate for the explanation of the season of birth findings". He suggested two possible types of evidence that would indicate etiological reasons for the excess of winter births in schizophrenia: (1) the existence of a stronger degree of association in a specific subset of schizophrenic patients, and (2) the existence of results tied to a precise etiological hypothesis. A viral hypothesis, for example, predicts that the association of season of birth with schizophrenia would be stronger in non-familial rather than familial schizophrenics: the evidence on this point is equivocal, however, as is shown below.

Several researchers have examined the effect of temperature as a possible cause of the seasonal variation in births. Pasamanick (1986) suggested that the winter excess of births of schizophrenic patients may be a result of the effect of hot summers on gestation, but studies in Sweden (McNeil et al., 1975), the United Kingdom (Hare & Moran, 1981), and Minnesota, USA (Watson et al., 1984) have failed to find an association between the winter birth rate and temperatures in the previous summer or autumn. Hare & Moran (1981), however, found an association between cold winters and births of schizophrenic patients in England, and an analysis of data from the Scottish Psychiatric Case Register (Kendell & Adams, 1991) indicated that an elevated incidence of schizophrenic births in the late winter and spring is related to low mean monthly temperatures six months previously, in the autumn. It is possible that a nutritional, infectious or other factor associated with cool weather could exert an effect in the second trimester of fetal development.

Müller & Kleider (1990), analysing data on nearly 9000 births in the Federal Republic of Germany between 1967 and 1971, showed that premature births were more common in March. They suggested that minimal brain damage associated with premature delivery could produce a seasonal excess of births of people with schizophrenia or other brain disorders. Häfner et al. (1987), in fact, reported a winter excess of births, not only in schizophrenia, but also for mental retardation, depression and bipolar disorder, all of which might, theoretically, be increased in those born prematurely.

Maternal age is strongly correlated with various obstetric complications. Dalén (1990) pointed out that schizophrenic patients tend to be born to women with an elevated maternal age, and that births to older women, according to data from Denmark, Sweden and the United Kingdom, are more likely to occur in the early months of the year. Maternal age, he suggested, could explain the link between schizophrenia and winter births. Any neurodevelopmental hypothesis, including obstetric causes, would gain support if it were determined that the winter excess of schizophrenic births were confined to patients without a family history of mental disorder. As noted above, however, the findings on this point are equivocal. Studies that examined family history and season of birth are fairly evenly divided between those that confirm and those that reject this suggestion (Pulver et al., 1992). For example, one recent study (O'Callaghan et al., 1991) found that only schizophrenic patients without a family history for the illness demonstrated an excess of winter births, while another (Pulver et al., 1992) found the reverse—that schizophrenic patients born in the months of February to May had a stronger family history of schizophrenia.

A recent study in Milan, Italy (Sacchetti et al., 1992), provided evidence for a neurodevelopmental effect producing the excess of winter births among schizophrenics. A large number of patients with schizophrenia and major affective disorder were assessed for signs of brain damage by computerized tomography (CT). Patients with schizophrenia born between December and April were more likely to have signs of ventricular enlargement (but not cortical atrophy), and the abnormality was most common in those with no family history of the disorder. The findings were specific for schizophrenia; there was no association between birth date and ventricular enlargement in patients with affective disorder.

Maternal infection during gestation has been studied by several researchers as a possible neurodevelopmental cause for the seasonal fluctuation in schizophrenic births. Watson et al. (1984) reported an association between the annual incidence of births of schizophrenic patients and the incidence of diphtheria, pneumonia and influenza in Minnesota between 1916 and 1958. Torrey et al. (1988) found an association between births of schizophrenic subjects in Connecticut and Massachussetts and the reported rates of measles and varicella, but not influenza. Mednick et al. (1987) found an increased risk of schizophrenia among individuals who were in the second trimester of fetal development during the 1957 influenza epidemic in Helsinki, Finland. In a similar study of eight health regions in England and Wales (O'Callaghan et al., 1991), the number of schizophrenic patients born five months after the peak of the 1957 influenza epidemic was 88% higher than the average number of such births for the corresponding period in the two previous and two successive years. In Scotland, however, national data revealed no increased risk of schizophrenia associated with the 1918, 1919 or 1957 influenza epidemics (Kendell & Kemp, 1989). In the United States of America, a ten-state study failed to find an increase in schizophrenic births associated with the 1957 influenza epidemic (Bowler & Torrey, 1990), and in the Netherlands Selten & Slaets (1994) found no correlation between exposure to the epidemic in the second trimester and subsequent development of schizophrenia. However, Barr et al. (1990) established that higher than average rates of influenza, occurring in the sixth month of gestation, were associated with an elevated incidence of schizophrenic births in Denmark. Takei et al. (unpublished data) studied a sample of schizophrenic patients born in Denmark between 1915 and 1970, and established that exposure to influenza in utero was associated with an increased risk of schizophrenia. The number of babies who subsequently developed schizophrenia rose by 12% for every 100 000 cases of influenza in the general population in the sixth month of gestation. In a recent study of schizophrenic patients and influenza epidemics between 1939 and 1960 in England and Wales, Sham et al. (1992) found that exposure to influenza between the third and seventh month of gestation was associated with schizophrenia in adult life. Takei et al. (1994), using data from a large cohort of patients born in England and Wales between 1938 and 1965, found that females, but not males, exposed to influenza epidemics 5 months before birth had a significantly greater rate of schizophrenia as adults.

It is widely held that respiratory viral infections are frequently brought into the home by young children. To test the prediction that the risk of schizophrenia is lower in first-born children, and increased in individuals who had siblings of a young age while *in utero*, Sham et al. (1993) analysed data from a Swedish family study. Their results are consistent with these predictions. In particular, having siblings aged 3–4 years was associated with a significantly increased risk of schizophrenia, even after allowing for birth order, total number of siblings, and other potential confounders. The authors point out that these results, if replicated, could provide indirect support for the maternal viral infection hypothesis.

One of the most recent reports on this topic to date (Adams et al., 1993)—an analysis of Danish, English and Scottish data—is of particular interest since the researchers included some who had previously come to negative conclusions about the effect of maternal viral infection. The study found that exposure to the 1957 influenza epidemic in mid-pregnancy was associated with an increased incidence of schizophrenia, at least in female offspring, in all three countries. The effect appears to have been greatest in the fourth and sixth months of pregnancy. They also confirmed Sham et al.'s finding of a long-term association between season of birth and exposure to influenza in mid-pregnancy (in this case, in the sixth and seventh months) in England, but could find no such relationship in the Danish and Scottish data. The authors concluded that "despite several other negative studies ... maternal influenza during the middle third of intrauterine development, or something closely associated with it, is implicated in the etiology of some cases of schizophrenia".

There are a number of difficulties inherent in this area of research (Mednick et al., 1987). For example, there is generally no direct evidence that the subject's mother suffered a viral infection; the studies usually rely on hospital diagnosis; and the determination of stage of gestation at the time of exposure to the epidemic is based on date of birth. The infant may have had a pre-term or post-term delivery, however, and exposure may have occurred outside the official epidemic "window". One study that did derive direct evidence proved negative. The British perinatal mortality survey (Crow & Done, 1992) examined perinatal records and subsequent psychiatric hospital admissions for everyone born in England, Scotland and Wales in the week of 3–9 March 1958, a few months after the 1957 influenza epidemic. The offspring of 945 mothers who were known to have suffered from influenza in the second trimester of pregnancy failed to show an increased risk of developing schizophrenia.

Mednick et al. (1987) concluded that the viral effect may be one of many potential perturbations of gestation. They suggested that it may be less the type than the timing of the disturbance during fetal neural development that is critical in determining the risk of schizophrenia.

If an association between maternal viral infection and the subsequent development of schizophrenia is confirmed, it would point towards a number of etiological possibilities. Exposure to a virus could interfere with the process of cell migration in the fetal brain, it could produce a post-infectious encephalitis with a latency of 15 years or more, or it could predispose the individual to the later development of an autoimmune disease (Torrey et al., 1988). It is also possible that some unidentified infectious agent with a periodicity similar to the viral infection is responsible, or that the drugs used by the mother to combat the infection produce an effect on the fetus (Beiser & Iacono, 1990).

If season of birth variation is the result of a neurodevelopmental effect, the birth date will be associated with differences in age of onset, course and outcome of schizophrenia. A recent study, however, using data from two sources (the Edinburgh Psychiatric Case Register and the psychiatric in-patient records of the Scottish Health Service), and comparing two large populations of schizophrenic patients born in winter (January–March) and in summer (June–October) failed to find any evidence of such associations (Kendell & Kemp, 1987). Although there was a 9% excess of schizophrenic births in the first three months of the year among the Scottish patients, there were no detectable differences between patients born in winter or in summer in age of onset, sex ratio or prognosis.

The study of season of birth has proved to be a valuable area of research and may, eventually, uncover a risk factor which is relevant in a significant proportion of cases of schizophrenia.

3.2.7 Prevalence in different socioeconomic groups

In developed countries, schizophrenia and other mental disorders are more common in the lower socioeconomic groups. Faris & Dunham (1939) found that the highest prevalence rates for treated schizophrenia were concentrated in Chicago's poorer districts. From a rate of 7 per 1000 adults in the inner-city areas, the prevalence of treated schizophrenia declined gradually through the more affluent sections of the city to the lowest rates of below 2.5 per 1000 adults in the most prosperous areas. A number of other studies have confirmed that high rates of mental disorder, particularly schizophrenia, are concentrated in central low-income districts of many American and European cities (Schroeder, 1942; Gerard & Houston, 1953; Gardner & Babigian, 1966; Klee et al., 1967; Sundby & Nyhus, 1963; Hare, 1956). Schizophrenic patients in Nottingham, England, who took part in the WHO study of determinants of outcome (Giggs & Cooper, 1987) were found to be concentrated in central urban areas of low socioeconomic status.

Clark (1949) demonstrated that Chicago residents in low-income occupations had a higher incidence of treated schizophrenia than workers of higher status. This observation has been confirmed in a number of studies. In a survey in New Haven, Connecticut, Hollingshead & Redlich (1958) found a gradient of progressively greater prevalence of treated schizophrenia in the lower socioeconomic groups. The prevalence of illness was eleven times greater in the lowest group than in the highest. Ödegaard (1956) demonstrated that first admissions for schizophrenia to all psychiatric hospitals in Norway were most common among workers of low status, such as ordinary seamen and farm labourers, and one-third as frequent among owners and managers of businesses and other high-status occupations. In London, Stein (1957) demonstrated a social-class gradient for the incidence and prevalence of mental illness, with the highest rates in the lowest classes; the gradient was particularly evident for schizophrenia. Eaton (1985), in reviewing the data, concluded that, using three basic categories of social class, it is common to find a three-to-one difference in rates between the lowest and the highest classes.

Three principal explanations could account for the high rates of this illness in the poorer groups. The *social drift* (or social selection) theory suggests that people who are in the early stages of schizophrenia drift down to a lower social class as a result of their mental impairment. The *social stress* (or social causation) hypothesis proposes that the social stresses of poverty, deprivation and social disorganization increase the risk of developing schizophrenia. Finally, a *neurodevelopmental* explanation, which has been advanced to explain the high incidence of schizophrenia among immigrants in the United Kingdom (Eagles, 1991b), may also apply to the social-class gradient: lower-class members of the population may encounter more neurodevelopmental risk from obstetric complications, perinatal infection and other factors. The neurodevelopmental hypothesis is a variant of the social causation theory.

The neurodevelopmental hypothesis derives support from the evidence that obstetric complications are significantly associated with subsequent development of schizophrenia (Jacobsen & Kinney, 1980; Parnas et al., 1982; Lewis & Murray, 1987; Eagles et al., 1990) and that, in the United States of America particularly, infant mortality rates (an indicator of poor prenatal and obstetric care) are substantially higher among the poor.

Dohrenwend and co-workers (1992) demonstrated a social-class gradient for the prevalence of schizophrenia in Israel, with higher rates among the less well educated. However, they argue that the effect could not have a social causation because lower rates of schizophrenia were found among the more disadvantaged Israelis of North African background than among those of European background. Other factors, however, such as higher death rates among the disabled or culture-specific protective effects, may explain the lower rate of schizophrenia in north African Israelis.

Support for the social drift theory comes from a study conducted by Goldberg & Morrison (1963) in the United Kingdom which demonstrated that, although schizophrenic males were over-represented in the lowest socio-economic class, the social class of their fathers and other male family members was distributed much as in the general population. Similar findings have come from studies conducted in the USA (Turner & Wagenfeld, 1967).

A more recent study in the United Kingdom (Jones et al., 1993) confirmed that schizophrenic patients often fail to achieve the same occupational status as their fathers before the onset of illness, and also revealed that a similar effect did not occur in patients with affective psychosis. The underachieving schizophrenic patients also had poorer educational qualifications than the other schizophrenic subjects despite similar IQ scores before illness, a finding that suggests a developmental effect.

The social drift theory encounters difficulty in explaining the observation that the social-class gradient for the occurrence of schizophrenia is not usually observed in rural areas and is in fact inverted in the developing world. The link between schizophrenia and social class has been conclusively demonstrated only for city populations; the relationship is strongest in large cities and weaker in small cities and most rural areas. In the small town of Hagerstown, Maryland, for example, the prevalence of schizophrenia was not found to be related to social class (Kohn, 1973) and the same is true for Jaco's (1960) study of the state of Texas. At least nine studies conducted in India over the past 50 years (Elnagar et al., 1971; Dube & Kumar, 1972; Nandi et al., 1980; Torrey, 1987) have demonstrated that the prevalence of schizophrenia is greater in the higher castes than among the lower castes. Such a pattern cannot be explained by social drift, but could result from a higher death rate or recovery rate among schizophrenic individuals in the lower castes.

Two studies conducted 15 years apart in China (Province of Taiwan) in 1946–48 (Lin, 1953) and in 1961–63 (Lin et al., 1969), before and after a period of rapid industrial development, revealed a switch from one pattern of occurrence of schizophrenia to another. In the earlier study, the prevalence pattern for schizophrenia was found to be similar to that described for India, with higher rates being observed in the better-educated groups. In the second study, the prevalence gradient shifted to resemble that found in the industrial world. As Table 6 shows, the change is due to a decrease in the very high rates among the well-educated upper-class population observed in the earlier study. Since prevalence rates in the lower classes were not higher in the second study, the change in the pattern is not a result of reduced death rates or recovery rates in the lower classes.

The reason for the high prevalence rates among higher-caste Indians and the well-educated in the earlier Taiwanese study is not clear. They cannot be due to social drift: people cannot change their caste, nor would they "drift" into higher education. Many of the studies were field surveys and, therefore, would not be influenced by differences between groups in treatment-seeking behaviour. Changes in fetal and neonatal health, however, could produce a neuro-developmental effect. Improvements in neonatal care, in the early phase of industrialization, are likely to become available first to the better-off. Such a bias would increase the tendency for children born with obstetric complications in higher-class families to survive infancy with brain damage and for similar lower-class children to die early in life. This, in turn, would lead to higher rates of schizophrenia in the higher socioeconomic groups. If the later phase of industrial development brought advances in obstetric care selectively to the upper classes, this would eventually lead to *lower* rates of brain damage and a subsequent decrease in the incidence of schizophrenia in the upper classes.

This effect could be compounded by the influence of nutritional changes on the rate of obstetric complications in different groups in developing countries. For example, a significant proportion of women with poor nutrition have delivery complications as a result of pelvic contraction from childhood rickets.

55

Table 6

Prevalence of schizophrenia in China (Province of Taiwan) 1946-48 and 1961-63[a]

	Prevalence per 1000 population	
	1946-48	1961-63
Social class		
Upper	3.5	0.8
Middle	1.2	1.1
Lower	4.5	2.1
Occupation		
Professional	0.0	0.0
Merchant	3.6	0.9
Salaried worker	0.9	0.4
Labourer	1.7	1.9
Farmer, fisherman	1.7	1.1
Unemployed	3.8	5.5
Education		
College	18.2	0.0
Senior high school	13.0	1.9
Junior high school	5.7	0.0
Elementary education	1.1	1.2
No formal education	3.8	3.7

[a]Data from Lin et al. (1969).

Improvements in nutrition during industrial development reach the better-off groups first, but the first generation of women who gain this benefit are likely to be relatively small in stature and have a high rate of pelvic deformity. Their children, however—the first generation to have better nutrition from the outset—are bigger. Consequently, this first generation of more affluent women will have relatively small pelvic dimensions and will carry large, well nourished fetuses. The result is likely to be more difficult deliveries and more brain damage in the new generation of infants (Warner, 1994).

It is also possible that the early period of industrialization exerts unusual labour-market stresses on the better-educated workers. There may be a gradual switch from initial high levels of employment-related stress among the higher groups, who are more involved in the newly formed wage-labour force, to greater stress on the lower socioeconomic groups who become increasingly affected by poor work conditions, unemployment, poverty and deprivation. Such social and economic stresses, if they were to trigger the onset of schizophrenia, might produce a pattern of incidence in which the better-off are initially more severely afflicted and then less so (Warner, 1985).

Research conducted by Link et al. (1986) supports the possibility that adverse working conditions are a risk factor for schizophrenia. The researchers found that the first full-time jobs of people who subsequently developed schizophrenia were more likely to have had stressful features, such as hazards, fumes and extremes of humidity, heat, cold and noise, than the first jobs of community controls or patients suffering from depression. This finding could not be accounted for by downward social mobility in the schizophrenic group.

To summarize, several class-related factors acting with different force in different areas appear to produce the observed patterns of prevalence for schizophrenia. Social drift is almost certainly an important factor in urban industrial populations: neurodevelopmental effects and social stress may have an impact more broadly around the world.

3.2.8 Other risk factors

Urban residence

A number of studies indicate that schizophrenia is less common among rural than urban residents. The incidence of treated schizophrenia is consistently higher in urban areas than in rural districts, though this may be because rural dwellers are less likely to seek treatment or because people with schizophrenia and pre-schizophrenic features tend to drift towards urban centres (Eaton, 1974). Nevertheless, a recent study in Stockholm County, Sweden (Borgå, unpublished information), which used a broad-based sampling method, including general practitioners, prisons and social welfare offices, found a steep prevalence gradient for functional psychosis from rural, through suburban to the urban area. This finding suggests that the urban/rural gradient is not attributable to differences in participation in treatment.

Another recent study (Lewis et al., 1992), which looked at the association between place of upbringing and the incidence of schizophrenia among nearly 50 000 Swedish conscripts, argued against the possibility that schizophrenic individuals tend to drift into cities because of the illness or its prodrome. The researchers found that the incidence of schizophrenia was 1.65 times greater among men brought up in cities than in those who had a rural upbringing. Various environmental factors, therefore, may contribute to the urban concentration of schizophrenia: these include life-event stress and neurological damage from viral infection or childhood head trauma, all of which are more common in cities.

Marital status

Marital status has been found to be associated with risk of schizophrenia in several studies. The increased risk for unmarried as compared with married people ranges between 2.6 and 7.2; five studies reported an increased risk of 3.0–4.7 (Eaton, 1985). Women tend to marry earlier than men and to have a later onset of schizophrenia. It has been suggested that marriage exerts a protective effect which delays the onset of the illness in women. Alternatively, the illness in its early stages may act as a barrier to marriage. Eaton (1975), using incidence data from the Maryland Psychiatric Case Register, and Riecher-Rössler et al. (1992) have concluded that the latter explanation is more likely.

Stress

It has long been suspected that stress plays an important part in the onset of schizophrenia. An early study by Brown & Birley (1968) found a substantially greater incidence of stressful life events of various degrees of severity in the three-week period before the onset of episodes of the disorder in schizophrenic patients compared with control subjects in the general population. Since then, several other studies have been conducted, some confirming the results obtained by Brown & Birley, some failing to demonstrate any significant excess of stressful life events in the weeks prior to the appearance of the disorder. Norman & Malla (1993) reviewed these studies and noted that, of 14 comparisons, 5 demonstrated higher levels of antecedent stress in schizophrenic subjects than in controls, while none showed more stress in control groups. Schizophrenics do not experience higher levels of stress before episodes of illness than other psychiatric patients. According to Norman & Malla, the majority of studies that have tracked schizophrenic patients over time (23 of 30 comparisons reported in eight studies) have demonstrated that episodes of illness are likely to be preceded by increased levels of stress.

These issues have recently been examined in the framework of the WHO Study on the Determinants of Outcome of Severe Mental Disorders. The study involved nine sites, five in developed countries and four in developing countries (Day et al., 1987). A modified version of the Life Events Interview was used to assess 386 patients; events were recorded for the three-month period preceding onset. Overall rates of life events from six of the nine sites were similar to each other and to rates reported in prior studies which have identified a relationship between stress and the onset of schizophrenia: 60–65% of patients with an acute onset of illness reported a stressful life event in the 2–3 weeks before the onset of illness. In the Indian and Nigerian centres, rates of stressful events were lower, yet these centres reported the highest number of very acute conditions. The findings, therefore, suggest that the acute benign psychoses seen in the developing world are not psychogenic in origin. The authors of this study emphasize that life-event stress is neither necessary nor sufficient for the onset of acute psychotic symptoms. They conclude that "stressful life events are part of the pool of causal factors found to be associated with the onset of schizophrenia".

Migration

Ödegaard's (1932) study of Norwegian immigrants to Minnesota established that the incidence of schizophrenia in this group was about twice as high as in demographically comparable groups in Norway. Many studies since Ödegaard's pioneering work have attempted to find out whether migration represents a risk factor in schizophrenia. The picture that emerges from these data is inconsistent: while some migrant groups continue to show very high rates of hospital admission for schizophrenia, other studies fail to show an excess.

It is possible that the nature of migration has changed and that the process of self-selection that operated previously is no longer a prominent factor. There is evidence to suggest, however, that the variation in incidence rates is a consequence of whether the migrant enters the new culture at a high or low social status. Those who encounter poverty and stress are routinely found to experience higher rates of psychotic illness (Warner, 1985). On the other hand a number of studies have indicated that immigrants who enter a new culture with a high status experience rates of hospitalization for schizophrenia which are lower than those of other immigrants and close to those for native-born residents (Cade & Krupinski, 1962; Halevi, 1963; Malzberg, 1969; Cochrane, 1977).

A recent review of admission rates for schizophrenia in the United Kingdom provides support for this explanation. Among the four largest migrant populations living in England, hospital admission rates are higher among those born in India, Pakistan or the Caribbean, but the Irish have rates comparable to the population of Ireland. The higher admission rates can be explained, to a large extent, by demographic and socioeconomic factors for those born in India and Pakistan and by adverse post-migration experiences among the Caribbean population (Cochrane & Bal, 1987).

A series of studies of Afro-Caribbeans in the United Kingdom unexpectedly observed that schizophrenia is more common in second-generation immigrants than in the first generation. This finding supports the conclusion that the elevation in schizophrenia rates may be explained by (a) obstetric complications secondary to changes in maternal nutrition and (b) improved fetal survival resulting from better perinatal care (as discussed in section 3.2.7). An increase in obstetric complications and infant survival in immigrant women would not contribute at all to the rate of the illness among the first generation but would affect their offspring. A study by Harrison et al. (1988) demonstrated that the incidence of carefully diagnosed schizophrenia among Afro-Caribbeans in Nottingham was at least six times greater than among the indigenous population and that the vast majority of patients were second generation. A study in Birmingham showed that the schizophrenia rate was substantially greater among Afro-Caribbeans born in the United Kingdom than among first-generation immigrants or non-Caribbeans (McGovern & Cope, 1987). A study of Afro-Caribbeans in south London (Wessely et al., 1991) confirmed that the risk of schizophrenia was substantially greater in second-generation immigrants.

The most recent study on this issue was in central Manchester, and surveyed psychiatric admissions, over a period of four years, of people of European, Afro-Caribbean, and Asian extraction, taking particular care to differentiate between first- and second-generation immigrants. Rates for both first admissions and re-admissions were greatest among Afro-Caribbeans; rates among those of Asian extraction were similar to those for Europeans, except for the 16–29-year age group, who had lower rates than Europeans. In the Afro-Caribbean group, the higher rates were largely due to increased rates of schizophrenia; the highest rate occurred in second-generation Afro-Caribbeans (born in the United Kingdom) and was nine times that in Europeans (Thomas et al., 1993). The implication of these observations is that immigration itself does not increase the risk of schizophrenia: it is being born in the new country that is associated with increased hazards. An increased rate of maternal viral infection in the host country (Gupta, 1993), obstetric factors, or changing immunological responses could explain the increased risk to second-generation immigrants.

Seasonal variation

There is evidence of a seasonal variation in rates of admission to hospital for schizophrenia, with a peak in late spring and early summer (Hare, 1988). This seasonality has been observed in a number of countries over the past 180 years, but there appears to be no clear explanation for it.

Co-occurring disorders

Some illnesses appear to be less common among people with schizophrenia than in the general population: an example is rheumatoid arthritis and related conditions. In a review of 14 epidemiological studies carried out on this subject between 1934 and 1985, Eaton et al. (1992) found that the median prevalence rate of rheumatoid arthritis among schizophrenic subjects was 0.47%, significantly lower than the expected 1–3%. Three of the studies had reported a strong inverse relationship between the two disorders. A number of explanations for this finding have been proposed, including nutritional, hormonal, psychosocial, genetic and immunological mechanisms; autoimmune theories appear to be especially worthy of further investigation.

Many studies have shown that mortality is greater in schizophrenic patients: the increased death rate is seen for most causes of death, with the exception of cancer. Some researchers have suggested that cancer occurs less often in schizophrenic patients but this has not been proved (Gulbinat et al., 1992). Of particular interest is a study from Ireland conducted by Masterson & O'Shea (1984) which revealed that, although smoking is heavier and more than twice as common in schizophrenic patients than in the general population, the risk of lung cancer in the patient group is no greater. A recent WHO multi-site record-linkage study (Gulbinat et al., 1992) similarly showed that the risk of lung cancer was significantly lower for a large sample of schizophrenic patients in Denmark and was not elevated for schizophrenics in Hawaii, USA, and in Nagasaki, Japan. These findings suggest the possibility of a linkage in schizophrenia to a lung cancer suppressant gene or of an anti-tumour effect of phenothiazines (used in the treatment of schizophrenia). Concern has been expressed that elevated serum prolactin resulting from the use of phenothiazines may increase the risk of breast cancer in female patients: findings on this point have been inconsistent. The WHO multi-site study found no increased risk for patients in Denmark but did find an increased risk of breast cancer in Hawaii and Nagasaki, which gives cause for continued concern.

3.3 Epidemiological studies in primary health care facilities

Few studies have assessed the prevalence of schizophrenia in primary care settings. In one of the first studies, Parkes et al. (1962) found that more than

70% of a sample of schizophrenic patients discharged from London mental hospitals saw their general practitioner at least once in the following year: over half were seen more than five times. Retrospective surveys have found that 2% of primary care patients suffer from long-term mental illness: it is likely that the majority of these were schizophrenic.

Prospective studies have found an uneven distribution. Shepherd et al. (1966), studying a number of general practices, found that among some 15000 patients at risk during a twelve-month period, 0.6% had a diagnosis of psychosis. Using a two-stage assessment methodology, Schulberg et al. (1985) administered the DIS to 294 primary care patients; only one patient (0.3%) received a diagnosis of schizophrenia.

In a small town in Germany, Dilling (1980) found that four subjects (0.3%), out of a total of 1231 assessed by primary physicians during one year, were diagnosed as suffering from schizophrenia; the same number was found by a research interviewer.

Among 2743 patients who consulted a general practitioner in the course of a year, a psychiatric morbidity prevalence rate of 7% was found (Casey et al., 1984). Of these patients, schizophrenia was diagnosed (using the PSE) in 13% by the general practitioner and in 12% by the research interviewer; using the CATEGO diagnostic system the rate was 5%.

A survey in Salford, United Kingdom, in 1984 found that, whereas 75% of a group of 557 identified schizophrenic patients were in contact with psychiatrists, only seven were solely in contact with a general practitioner in the course of the year (Bamrah et al., 1991). The seven patients had been seen by psychiatrists in the past. The proportion in contact with a general practitioner alone was substantially smaller than in 1974. Despite the recent emphasis on community care in the United Kingdom, it appears that the care of schizophrenic patients is still overwhelmingly the responsibility of hospital-based psychiatric personnel.

In a survey of 369 general practitioners in the United Kingdom, 110 declared that the discharge of adult long-term mentally ill patients has had an effect on their practices (Kendrick et al., 1991). Most (225) estimated that they had 10 or fewer such patients on their list. Having higher numbers was significantly associated with practising in Greater London or within 5 km of a large mental hospital and having contact with a psychiatrist who visited the practice.

It is difficult to provide a precise figure for the proportion of general practice patients who suffer from schizophrenia. Several variables, including the availability of health and mental health services, the distance from a mental hospital, the extent of the deinstitutionalization process, and links between general practices and psychiatric services, can affect this rate. The likelihood of patients discharged from mental health facilities becoming linked to general practices may indeed be increased, or there may be a reporting bias, resulting from increased awareness of patients by the general practitioners. Patients with schizophrenia have been found to consult their general practitioner more often than the average patient, though no more often than those with chronic physical disorders (Nazareth et al., 1993). In inner city areas, lack of appropriate social networks may cause discharged mentally ill patients to have more contact with their general practitioners, thereby raising the doctor's level of awareness.

The only available data for the developing countries are those obtained by a WHO collaborative study carried out among 1624 patients attending primary health facilities in four countries (Colombia, India, Philippines and Sudan). The patients were assessed in a two-stage procedure, using a screening instrument followed by the PSE; a schizophrenia prevalence of 3.1% was found (Harding et al., 1980).

3.4 Epidemiological studies in psychiatric facilities

As might be expected, people with schizophrenia are over-represented in psychiatric institutions as compared with the rate found in the community or in primary care settings. For instance, in the United States, on a selected day in 1986, there were a total of 69994 inpatients in psychiatric facilities with a primary diagnosis of schizophrenia, corresponding to 43.5% of all psychiatric inpatients on that date. This was the largest diagnostic group: the second largest, those with affective disorders, accounted for 21.6% of the total (Manderscheid & Sonnenschein, 1990).

Considerable differences in the relative frequency of these two major diagnostic groupings were found in the different types of facilities. In state and county mental hospitals, Veterans' Administration medical centres, and multiservice mental health organizations, schizophrenia was the most frequent diagnosis (58%, 41% and 44%, respectively). In private psychiatric hospitals and non-federal general hospitals, affective disorders were most common (50% and 37%, respectively).

In 1980 there were 369402 admissions with a primary diagnosis of schizophrenia (23% of all psychiatric admissions). Again, schizophrenia was more common among people admitted to state and county mental hospitals, Veterans' Administration medical centres and multiservice mental health organizations. Because they tend to stay longer in hospital, people with schizophrenia comprised a much higher percentage of the population under care than of those admitted. The median length of inpatient stay for people with a diagnosis of schizophrenia was 19 days; the median stay was longer for those who were inpatients in state and county mental hospitals (38 days).

Among all psychiatric patients receiving outpatient care on the census day in 1986, there were 298808 people (21.6% of the total) with a diagnosis of schizophrenia; approximately the same proportion had affective disorders (22.3%). In the same year 166737 people (7.8%) were admitted to outpatient care with a diagnosis of schizophrenia.

In Ireland, in 1988, the proportion of psychiatric patients diagnosed as suffering from schizophrenia was 180 per 100000 admissions and 33.8 per 100000 among first admissions (O'Connor & Walsh, 1991). The rate of schizophrenia among admissions was higher for males (210 per 100 000) than for females (149 per 100 000). Schizophrenia was most common among admissions in the age group 35–44 years and among unskilled manual workers. More than half of the patients admitted with such a diagnosis stayed in hospital less than one month.

3.5 Epidemiological studies in other facilities or among special population groups

3.5.1 Prisoners

One review of the literature concluded that 6–8% of the 147 000 inmates of local jails in the United States of America in the 1970s were psychotic (Warner, 1985). People with psychosis, however, accounted for only 2–5% of people admitted to jail, leading to the conclusion that the mentally ill were being detained longer than other offenders (Lamb & Grant, 1982).

Similarly, 8% of a large sample of federal prisoners in the USA surveyed in 1969 were diagnosed as psychotic (Roth & Ervin, 1971). A review of surveys carried out in prisons in the United Kingdom, on the other hand (Coid, 1984), concluded that psychoses (including schizophrenia) were not frequent, but highlighted the methodological limitations of many studies.

Three recent surveys employing reliable methodology have been carried out among prisoners. In Canada, Bland et al. (1990) used the DIS and other questionnaires to interview 180 randomly selected male prisoners aged 18–44 years. A comparison was made with 1006 similarly aged male residents of Edmonton who were interviewed using the same instruments. The prevalence rate for schizophrenia among the prisoners (2.2%) was substantially higher than the rate found in the community sample (0.6%).

In the USA, Teplin (1990) calculated the current and lifetime prevalence rates of schizophrenia among 627 male jail detainees interviewed with the DIS and compared them with those found in 3481 male subjects, aged 18–60 years, living in the community and included in the ECA sample. The author found a current prevalence rate for schizophrenia in the sample of detainees of 2.74% compared with 0.91% in the community sample: the lifetime prevalence rates were respectively 3.71% and 1.70%. The differences between the jail and general populations continued to be significant after controlling for race and age.

In the United Kingdom, Gunn et al. (1991) administered a semi-structured interview to a 5% sample of men serving prison sentences (404 young offenders and 1365 adults): 1.2% of the inmates were diagnosed as suffering from schizophrenia according to ICD-9 criteria. This rate is comparable to other prison surveys in the United Kingdom which used clinical criteria (Roger, 1950; Gunn et al., 1978). Although this prevalence rate is comparable to that found in the community, it nevertheless represents a considerable problem given the limited array of therapeutic options available in prisons.

3.5.2 The homeless

A review of published data suggests that, between 1960 and 1985, 25–50% of homeless men in large American cities suffered from a psychotic disorder. Among women the proportion was higher—by some estimates, 75–90% (Warner, 1985). In a recent review of eight studies published on this topic since 1984, with sample sizes ranging from 49 to 328 homeless people (Fischer & Breakey, 1991), lifetime prevalence rates of schizophrenia ranging from 1.4% to 30.3% were found. Two of these studies, with large samples and careful methodology, deserve particular mention.

Koegel et al. (1988) conducted a survey among 328 homeless people living in inner Los Angeles, using a version of the DIS modified to make it more sensitive for a homeless population. An overall lifetime prevalence of schizophrenia of 13.1% was found: this compares with a rate of 0.5% in the Los Angeles general community sample in the ECA study ($n = 3055$). The risk ratio for schizophrenia in the homeless sample compared with the community was 26:1. The lifetime prevalence rate was especially high among the long-term homeless (18%). The prevalence of schizophrenia among the homeless is, clearly, much higher than in the general population but, given the tendency of the DIS to produce a high number of false-positive results for schizophrenia, the prevalence figure in this study should be treated with caution.

In a sample of homeless people in Baltimore, USA (Breakey et al., 1989), 125 men and 78 women were examined by psychiatrists using the Standardized Psychiatric Examination. A schizophrenia prevalence rate of 12% among men and 17% among women was found; in addition, a high rate of comorbidity, especially of alcohol and substance abuse disorders, was detected in the sample. Finally, a recent study compared the prevalence of schizophrenia among the homeless residents of Edinburgh hostels in 1966 and 1992. Despite a 66% reduction in the number of beds available for psychiatric care of adults in the region during that period, the prevalence of schizophrenia among this homeless population was lower in 1992 (9%) than in 1966 (25%), even after other changes in the population were taken into account (Geddes et al., 1994).

3.6 Epidemiological research and the etiology of schizophrenia

3.6.1 Implications of neuroanatomical and neurophysiological research

Research on brain structure and function has advanced our understanding of the etiology of schizophrenia and has raised new questions that need to be addressed by epidemiological research. Post-mortem studies of schizophrenic patients have revealed degenerative changes in the limbic system, an area of the brain that is important in the regulation of emotion and response to stress; such changes are not found in non-schizophrenics (Averback, 1981; Stevens, 1982). In addition, over 50 studies using computerized tomographic (CT) scans have found evidence of mild cerebral atrophy in a proportion of schizophrenic patients (Van Horn & McManus, 1992). The changes, which include enlargement of the ventricles of the brain and widening of the cerebral fissures, also occur in degenerative brain conditions and in some other psychiatric patients (Weinberger & Kleinman, 1986).

The cause of cerebral atrophy in schizophrenia is not known. Since the abnormalities are found equally in "first-break" schizophrenics (those experiencing their first psychotic episode) and in chronic patients, it is unlikely that the changes are due to treatment. The atrophy does not indicate that schizophrenia is a degenerative brain disease: it is not progressive, it is not specific to schizophrenia, and it is not present in all cases. The changes occur in only about a quarter of schizophrenic patients. There is no well defined group with enlarged cerebral ventricles: the changes seen on the CT scans are distributed along a continuum from normal to large (Weinberger & Kleinman, 1986). The most probable explanation is that the cerebral atrophy found in some schizophrenics is an indicator of earlier brain injury which increased the person's vulnerability to the illness. Such brain damage might result, for example, from the effects of drugs administered to the person's mother during pregnancy, maternal viral illness, birth trauma, postnatal infection or a similar assault. It will be important to establish which, if any, of these factors is, in fact, associated with an increased risk of schizophrenia. The perinatal mortality survey in the United Kingdom (Done et al., 1991) is an example of a well designed epidemiological study in which relationships were sought between multiple perinatal risk factors and the subsequent development of a variety of psychiatric conditions in a nationwide sample of births during a single week.

Changes seen on CT scans are not restricted to one clinical subtype of the illness, but schizophrenic patients with these signs of brain damage have some characteristic clinical features. Patients with evidence of cerebral atrophy have more severe negative symptoms of schizophrenia, such as apathy, withdrawal and poverty of ideas: positive symptoms, such as hallucinations and delusions, are less prominent. They are also more likely to display poor premorbid functioning, to show signs of neurological impairment, to respond poorly to medication and to have an unfavourable outcome (Weinberger & Kleinman, 1986). Crow (1980) suggested that schizophrenia could be classified as type 1, in which positive symptoms predominate, or type 2, in which negative symptoms are prominent; such subtyping may be useful in epidemiological research to evaluate the importance of neurodevelopmental risk factors.

It is likely that both inheritance and early brain damage are risk factors for schizophrenia. Studies of identical twins discordant for schizophrenia, for example, reveal that the affected twin is more likely to have a history of obstetric complications at birth (McNeil, 1987) and evidence of brain damage (as shown on CT scans, for example) (Reveley et al., 1982; Suddath et al., 1989). Epidemiological studies of the impact of both genetic loading and early brain damage (by evaluating the family history of psychosis and perinatal records) will be valuable in determining the extent to which these risk factors act independently or in concert. A recent study of this type from Sweden

(McNeil et al., 1993) found that head circumference was smaller in relation to body length in preschizophrenic infants than in controls. Small head size was associated with an absence of a family history of psychosis, suggesting a non-genetic cause, but was not related to season of birth or obstetric complications: thus, links to viral infection or birth trauma were not established.

Abnormalities of brain function in schizophrenia have also been described (Bloom, 1993). Some researchers have detected a "sensory gating" abnormality in the limbic system. Using computerized averaging of multiple electro-encephalograph tracings (evoked potentials), Freedman et al. (1991) measured differences between people from the general population, people with schizophrenia and their relatives in their response to repeated auditory and visual stimuli. The research showed that most schizophrenic patients, as well as half of their close relatives, were limited in their ability to screen out irrelevant information. Thus, the capacity to discriminate stimuli and to focus attention may be disrupted in those who are vulnerable to schizophrenia. Given sufficient stress, the affected individual may become aroused and hypervigilant or, as a defensive manoeuvre, withdrawn and autistic (Freedman et al., 1991).

The evidence that half of the first-degree relatives of schizophrenics share a neurophysiological abnormality with schizophrenics themselves suggests that the defect is genetically transmitted. The most recent work indicates that abnormal sensory gating in schizophrenia is linked to the gene that controls the function of brain nicotine receptors (Adler et al., 1992). This raises another question, however: why do only some of those with the defect develop schizophrenia? Recent research using magnetic resonance imaging reveals that in schizophrenics the hippocampus (part of the limbic system) is smaller than in healthy siblings who have the same sensory gating abnormality. It is possible that early damage to the hippocampus, combined with an inherited sensory gating defect, is sufficient to produce schizophrenia (Freedman et al., 1991). Measures of sensory gating (and, similarly, smooth-pursuit eye-movement abnormalities) may become increasingly valuable in tracing relatives of schizophrenics who are vulnerable to the illness.

More advanced brain-imaging techniques are uncovering an increasingly complex picture of functional abnormalities in schizophrenia. Research using radioactive tracer substances and positron emission tomography (PET) has demonstrated that blood flow through the frontal lobes of the brain does not increase in schizophrenic patients, as it does in other people, when they undertake tasks requiring attention and effort. People with schizophrenia may not be able to "turn on" a specific region of their frontal lobes, the prefrontal cortex, when needed—a problem that could explain the withdrawal, apathy and cognitive problems in schizophrenia (Franzen & Ingvar, 1975; Weinberger & Kleinman, 1986). The prefrontal cortex and the limbic system are linked: an abnormality in one could affect the other, though it is not certain which area is primarily disturbed (Weinberger & Kleinman, 1986). Drawing on the results of recent magnetic resonance imaging studies, Carpenter & Buchanan (1994) conclude that "limbic-system circuitry is involved in the pathophysiology of psychosis, and the dorsolateral prefrontal cortical circuitry in the pathophysiology of enduring negative symptoms".

Step by step, links are being forged between inheritance patterns, neurophysiological and anatomical abnormalities, environmental stress and the symptoms of schizophrenia. Epidemiological research that aims to tease out answers to questions of etiology must consider multiple factors—for example, gender, family history, possible genetic markers such as sensory gating deficits and smooth-pursuit eye-movement abnormalities, evidence of brain damage, attention difficulties, predominance of negative symptoms, and perinatal complications. An example of research that weighs the impact of several of these factors is the study by Sacchetti et al. (1992), cited in section 3.2.6, which evaluated the interactions of ventricular enlargement, season of birth, and family history for psychosis in patients with both schizophrenia and affective disorders.

3.6.2 Studies of high-risk groups

Schizophrenia is not a common disorder: consequently, it is expensive to study precursors of the illness in randomly selected community samples, since a large number of individuals are needed for meaningful statistical analyses to be done. For this reason, some prospective studies use "high-risk samples" in which children at increased risk of developing schizophrenia are identified before the onset of the disorder and are assessed over time. One goal of such research is to separate the antecedents of the disorder from its secondary deficits. These studies also provide an opportunity to investigate biological markers for genetic vulnerability to schizophrenia. In most cases, the offspring of people who suffer from schizophrenia are selected as subjects. A Danish project (Mednick et al., 1987), which started in 1962, examined 207 adolescents with schizophrenic mothers, and a group of control subjects. Another project was launched in New York, in 1971, by Erlenmeyer-Kimling & Cornblatt (1987a): they evaluated 355 children, aged 7–12 years, who were born to schizophrenic mothers, other hospitalized psychiatric patients or normal controls.

Asarnow (1988) reviewed 24 studies of high-risk groups and concluded that some high-risk children can be distinguished on the basis of neurointegrative problems, social impairment and early symptomatology. Such impairments generally become apparent in middle childhood and adolescence. Although some deficits are not specific for schizophrenia, deficits in attention and information processing, in neuromotor functions (particularly smooth-pursuit eye-movement), and in social behaviour may be specifically associated with increased risk for schizophrenia. In addition, some family attributes, including family communication deviance, negative affective style and a high level of criticism and intrusiveness (expressed emotion) are associated with a higher risk of schizophrenia. It is unclear, however, if these family attributes increase the risk of the illness or are merely a secondary response to premorbid problems of the pre-schizophrenic offspring.

4

Temporal trends

Some diseases are provoked by affluence and tend to grow with industrial progress: others are a response to poverty and tend to decrease in incidence with the advance of industrialization. A number of diseases associated with industrialization, however, are influenced both by affluence *and* poverty, and the incidence has been found to rise early in the process of development and to fall later. Like schizophrenia in China (Province of Taiwan) (see section 3.2.7), they are initially more common among the rich and, later, become more common among the poor. Such diseases include thyrotoxicosis, peptic ulcer, poliomyelitis, appendicitis and ischaemic heart disease (Barker, 1989). The reasons for the rise and fall in incidence vary from condition to condition but are often related to an environmental change in hygiene or diet which acts in childhood to modify the susceptibility of the individual, or to a particular factor exerting an effect later in life to produce illness. For example, people whose dietary iodine is deficient in youth are less able to adapt to an increase in iodine intake later in life and tend to develop thyrotoxicosis (Barker & Phillips, 1984).

Kraepelin, in 1926, described such a pattern of changing occurrence for general paralysis of the insane, pointing out that it "was formerly uncommon, underwent a progressively rapid increase from the beginning of the last century and for some time now has been gradually diminishing". A similar pattern for schizophrenia has been proposed by various researchers.

4.1 Was schizophrenia rare before the eighteenth century?

Torrey (1980) has suggested that schizophrenia may not have existed prior to the eighteenth century. This hypothesis has been rejected by a number of authors (Jeste et al., 1985; Ellard, 1987). Jeste cited evidence, for example, that the inhabitants of ancient India and Rome distinguished schizophrenia-like conditions from those resembling mania, depression, catatonic stupor and delirium. A more complex issue, however, is whether schizophrenia was less common before the eighteenth century.

Hare (1983) argued that there was a real increase in the occurrence of schizophrenia in the United Kingdom during the nineteenth century. Not only did the total number of people in asylums increase, but so did admission and first-admission rates. First admissions more than tripled between 1869 and 1900. As an editorial in the London *Times* of 1877 quipped, "if lunacy continues to increase as at present, the insane will be in the majority, and, freeing themselves, will put the sane in asylums" (Scull, 1979). Many of the asylum superintendents, caught, as it seemed, in an upward spiral of lunacy, were at pains to point out that this trend reflected increasing recognition of those in need of treatment, and was not an indictment of their attempts at prevention. Others, like Daniel Hack Tuke (1894), believed that there was an actual increase in mental disorder brought about by the spread of poverty. Hare (1983), following Tuke, argued that increased recognition of insanity cannot explain a sustained growth rate on such a scale over several decades. If increasing numbers of mild cases were being admitted to the asylums, he contended, one would expect to find decreasing death rates and increasing recovery rates, and this was not the case. Hare pointed out, moreover, that the greatest increase was in "melancholia", the condition that most closely matches the modern diagnosis of schizophrenia.

In a recent article, Hare (1988b) further developed the "recency hypothesis", arguing that the early-onset type of schizophrenia increased during the nineteenth century, accounting, at least in part, for the increase in diagnosed insanity. He suggested that some biological event (e.g., a viral mutation or a changed immunological reaction to existing infections) caused an increase in schizophrenia around 1800. In Hare's opinion, the recency hypothesis "provides a straightforward and consistent explanation for all the major aspects of the history and epidemiology of schizophrenia" (Hare, 1988b).

Even at the end of the nineteenth century, schizophrenia appears to have been relatively rare. Jablensky (1986) reported that only 9.1% of men and 7.3% of women, on first admission to the University Psychiatric Clinic in Munich in 1908, were diagnosed as suffering from dementia praecox. Since Kraepelin himself evaluated some of these cases, it is unlikely that missed diagnosis accounts for the low prevalence of the disorder among those admitted. The occurrence rate for the diagnostic categories most likely to have included schizophrenia was low among other nineteenth century asylum populations, Jablensky argues. The greatest increase in institutionalized cases of schizophrenia, he suggests, may well have occurred in the present century.

Some authors have pushed the study of this issue back to earlier times. In reviewing the treatment records of the English mediaeval physician, Richard Napier, Ellard (1987) concluded that the condition closest to our modern category of schizophrenia, namely "mopishness", was not a common condition. Though interesting, quantitative speculation based on such ancient records is crude at best.

The interpretation of historical prevalence data, moreover, faces the same difficulties as does the debate on the prevalence of schizophrenia in the present-day developing world. The low recorded rates, in each instance, may be a result of restricted access to treatment, high mortality, or rapid recovery of affected individuals. Although the prevalence of schizophrenia in developing societies appears to be lower than in the industrial world, the incidence of the disease is not. This observation suggests that we should exercise a similar degree of caution in evaluating historical treatment prevalence rates, since they may bear little relation to the actual occurrence of mental disorders.

4.2 Is the incidence of schizophrenia on the decline?

Der et al. (1990) have pointed out that the incidence of schizophrenia, as determined in several recent studies, appears to be on the decline. Studies that have examined changes in the incidence of schizophrenia since 1960 are listed in Table 7. The studies upon which Der and associates based their opinion are included in this table, as well as a number of other studies, some of which have appeared since the publication of their paper, that show no change or an increase in incidence. More than two-thirds of the studies listed in Table 7 indicate a decrease in the incidence of the illness since 1960. All of the studies relied upon service-contact data, either first-contact or first-admission, and the figures are age-standardized in only a few instances. A recent study found a decrease in the occurrence of schizophrenia in those born after 1940. Waddington & Youssef (1994) demonstrated that the morbid risk for men born between 1940 and 1969 in a small area of Ireland was 19% lower than the risk for men born between 1920 and 1939. The morbid risk for women decreased by 56% over the same time period.

It is possible that a diagnostic shift from schizophrenia to another diagnostic category could account for a decrease in the observed occurrence of schizophrenia (Strömgren, 1987; Crow, 1990). The switch between editions of the International Classification of Diseases, for example, may have narrowed the diagnosis of schizophrenia. The major ICD diagnostic shift took place in the late 1960s, but Gupta & Murray (1991) argue that the decrease in the incidence of schizophrenia began somewhat earlier, in the mid-1960s, in England and Scotland. Parker et al. (1985) found that the decrease in the incidence of treated schizophrenia in New South Wales, Australia, was accompanied by an increase in the diagnosis of affective psychosis following the introduction of lithium carbonate. Other studies (Dickson & Kendell, 1986; Eagles et al., 1988) have shown a similar increase in the prevalence of affective psychoses, though many have not.

A recent study by Kendell et al. (1993) strengthens the argument that the changing incidence of schizophrenia is an artefact, produced by a diagnostic shift. In a detailed study of the diagnoses attributed to a 50% sample of first admissions to psychiatric facilities in and around Edinburgh, Scotland, the researchers showed that the proportion diagnosed as schizophrenic by hospital psychiatrists decreased by 22% between 1971 and 1989. When diagnoses for these patients were made according to a computer algorithm, however, there was no such decline; in fact there was a small increase in the proportion diagnosed as having schizophrenia.

A comparison of diagnostic practices and longitudinal trends in the incidence of schizophrenia in France and the United Kingdom between 1973 and 1982 leads to the conclusion that diagnostic drift has occurred in opposite directions in the two countries producing a diverging incidence of the disease. In the United Kingdom, an increase in the use of standardized criteria may have led to an increase in the category of "other psychoses" and a decrease in schizophrenia. In France, the influence of Jacques Lacan and other psycho-

Table 7

Trends in the incidence of schizophrenia since 1960

Authors	Country or area	Period	Measure	Change in frequency
Eagles & Whalley (1985)	Scotland	1969–78	Age-standardized first-admission rate	40% decrease
Parker et al. (1985)	New South Wales, Australia	1967–77	Number of first admissions	9% decrease
Dickson & Kendell (1986)	Scotland	1970–81	Number of first admissions	48% decrease
Häfner & an der Heiden (1986)	Mannheim, Fed. Rep. of Germany	1963–80	First-contact rates	18% increase
Munk-Jørgensen (1986)	Denmark	1970–84	Age-standardized first-admission rates	37% decrease
Munk-Jørgensen & Jørgensen (1986)	Denmark	1970–84	Age-standardized first-admission rates	44% decrease (female)
Joyce (1987)	New Zealand	1974–84	Number of first admissions	37% decrease
Eagles et al. (1988)	Aberdeen, UK	1969–84	Age-standardized first-contact rates	54% decrease
de Alarcon et al. (1990)	Oxford, UK	1975–86	Age-standardized first-contact rates Age-standardized first-ever diagnosis rate	50% decrease (males & females)
Der et al. (1990)	UK	1970–86	First-admission rates	40% decrease (males) 50% decrease (females)
Folnegović et al. (1990)	Croatia	1965–84	First-admission rates	No change
Bamrah et al. (1991)	Salford, UK	1974–84	Age-standardized first-contact rates	64% increase
Castle et al. (1991)	Camberwell, UK	1965–84	Age-standardized first-contact rates	25% increase (ICD) 40% increase (RDC) 38% increase (DSM-III)
Harrison et al. (1991)	Nottingham, UK	1975–87	Age-specific first-contact rates	No change
Munk-Jørgensen & Mortensen (1992)	Denmark	1969–88	First-ever admission rates	50% decrease
Geddes et al. (1993)	Scotland	1969–88	First-ever admission rates	57% decrease (males) 43% decrease (females)

71

analysts produced a broadening of the concept of schizophrenia and an increase in diagnosed cases (van Os et al., 1993).

Problems surround the definition of "first admission" used in many studies because the diagnosis at the time of first contact or admission may change subsequently. In Denmark, only 50% of those eventually diagnosed as suffering from schizophrenia receive such a diagnosis at the time of their first admission. De Alarcon et al. (1990), however, found that the incidence of schizophrenia could be shown to have decreased in Oxford, England, for both first and subsequent diagnoses. Munk-Jørgensen (1987a, 1987b), similarly, determined that a decline in first-admission rates had occurred even when this factor was taken into account.

A substantial shift away from hospital treatment and towards community care has occurred since 1960 in many countries and this change may have resulted in fewer cases being included in traditional treatment-based statistics (Crow, 1990; Munk-Jørgensen & Mortensen, 1992). Some people with schizophrenia may never be admitted to hospital. It is of interest, therefore, that some estimates based on first contact with any type of psychiatric facility (as opposed to first hospital admission) also show a significant decrease in the incidence of schizophrenia (Eagles et al., 1988; de Alarcon et al., 1990; Kendell et al., 1993). Other first-contact-based studies, however, do not show such a decrease (Häfner & an der Heiden, 1986; Bamrah et al., 1991; Castle et al., 1991; Harrison et al., 1991).

It is likely that the increased use of antipsychotic drugs has led to a greater number of patients being treated successfully by general practitioners and, consequently, never being referred to any type of psychiatric treatment agency or included in service-based statistics (Graham, 1990; de Alarcon et al., 1990). Similarly, more psychotic people may escape any kind of treatment and, instead, live in seclusion as vagrants, in shelters for the homeless, or in jail. An incidence study of schizophrenia in Nottingham, England (Cooper et al., 1987), for instance, found that 10% of the cases that were ultimately detected were missed in the original screening as they were only fleetingly in contact with the treatment facilities. Further cases with no contact at all with the formal psychiatric treatment system (who may have seen a general practitioner, for example) would have escaped detection altogether. The size of the population that remains undetected and the extent to which it may have increased in recent years is not known, but could be considerable.

Migration and changes in the age structure of the population could account for changes in the incidence of schizophrenia. Several of the studies indicating a decrease in incidence, however, use age-standardized statistics, and a number use statistics for an entire country or region, which makes an effect of migration unlikely. On the other hand, an apparent increase in the incidence of schizophrenia in Camberwell, England, has been attributed to migration. Afro-Caribbean residents of Camberwell show rates of schizophrenia six times that of other ethnic groups and, it is argued, the increase in the proportion of this immigrant population in the area may account for the high local rate of the illness (Castle et al., 1991). The same argument could be used to explain the stable or increasng schizophrenia rates in Nottingham and Salford, England.

The recent findings of decreasing admission rates for schizophrenia since the 1960s are thrown into doubt by long-term studies, presenting data that do not indicate a decreasing trend. Häfner (1987) reviewed nine studies, which reported changes in the morbid risk of schizophrenia over periods ranging from 38 to 130 years. Among the nine studies, three, using data from two countries, were methodologically more sophisticated and deserve special attention. Using the Norwegian National Case Register, Ödegaard (1971) investigated all first admissions for schizophrenia over a period of 40 years, later extended to 63 years by Astrup (1982), and found that the rates varied little, ranging from an initial value of 0.18/0.19 per 1000 (male/female) in 1916 to a final value of 0.20/0.25 per 1000 in 1978. Krupinski & Alexander (1983) studied all admissions for schizophrenia to the psychiatric hospitals of the State of Victoria, Australia, over 130 years (1848–1978). They checked the diagnoses given by retrospectively applying DSM-III criteria to randomly selected samples of patients, each consisting of 100 admissions in successive periods of time. They found a fairly stable age-corrected admission rate for schizophrenia.

Other reviews conclude that the case for the declining incidence of schizophrenia is so far unproved, but merits further investigation (Castle, 1993; Harrison & Mason, 1993; Jablensky, 1993). If there is, in fact, any true decrease in the incidence of schizophrenia, the finding could be of considerable etiological significance. Possible explanations for the phenomenon include a decrease in the fertility of people with schizophrenia, a reduction in social or economic stress, a change in the herd immunity to a causative infectious agent, and a decrease in neurodevelopmental risk factors resulting from improvements in obstetric care.

To produce a decrease in the incidence of schizophrenia throughout the 1970s, it would be necessary for a change in the fertility of schizophrenics to have occurred through the 1950s. With the decrease in the use of hospital confinement for the mentally ill, however, a movement that began in many countries in the mid-1950s, it is probable that the trend has been more towards increased fertility in schizophrenics, rather than a decrease. The fertility of schizophrenic patients, moreover, is unlikely to play a large part in the observed decline in the incidence of the illness because, as noted above, only 11% of people with schizophrenia have a schizophrenic parent.

As mentioned above, the early stages of industrialization may produce high levels of employment-related stress which afflicts first the better-off groups and later the lower classes. In the modern late-industrial societies in which the decline in the incidence of schizophrenia is being noted, however—Australia, Denmark and the United Kingdom—unemployment and poverty are not on the decline. It is difficult, therefore, to see how economic and social trends can have led to a decline in illness rates.

Increased rates of immunization and improvements in hygiene have produced changes in herd immunity to various infectious agents. Poliomyelitis, for example, increased in prevalence with industrialization as a result of changes in immunity. In this instance, vulnerability of the central nervous system to poliovirus infection increases with age. As hygiene and sanitation improved, the proportion of children escaping infection during the relatively safe period of infancy increased, and the number of cases of paralytic disease rose in parallel, affecting the higher socioeconomic groups first (Barker, 1989). The prevalence of poliomyelitis subsequently declined in developed countries as a result of immunization programmes. Similar changes in immunity or exposure to viral infection might account for the reported changes in the prevalence of schizophrenia over time and within social groups.

Developments in obstetric practice may similarly account for the observed changes in the incidence of schizophrenia. The relative risk of schizophrenia in people with obstetric complications compared with those without has been estimated to be 2.5:1 (Goodman, 1988). The decline in early neonatal mortality rates in England and Wales was paralleled by the subsequent fall in the first-admission rate for schizophrenia in the 1960s and 1970s (Gupta & Murray, 1991).

Obstetric factors could explain why decreases in the incidence of schizophrenia in the United Kingdom have been greatest in the most prosperous regions (Gupta & Murray, 1991), why the districts that show no decrease in schizophrenia have large immigrant populations with high rates of poverty (Eagles, 1991b), and why schizophrenia rates in developed countries are higher among the poor. Afro-Caribbean infants in the United Kingdom (Terry et al., 1987; Griffiths et al., 1989) and black infants in the United States of America (North & MacDonald, 1977) are more likely to be of low birth weight, but have higher survival rates than white infants of low birth weight. Since some studies have found that schizophrenic patients tend to have lower birth weights than their healthy siblings (Lane & Albee, 1966; Stabenau & Pollin, 1967), it is possible that intrauterine development and survival may contribute to the high risk of schizophrenia in lower social groups and among immigrants.

4.3 Changes in the clinical picture of schizophrenia

Although there is controversy over the question of a decline in the incidence of schizophrenia, most authors agree that a substantial change has occurred in the clinical picture of the illness in the course of this century, with a marked decrease in the occurrence of catatonic schizophrenia in developed countries (Leff, 1988). A similar decline has not been seen in most developing countries, particularly in Africa, where catatonic forms of schizophrenia are still quite common (Odejide et al., 1989). The proportion of hebephrenic cases has also decreased in developed countries, whereas the number of paranoid and undifferentiated cases has increased (Hare, 1988a).

Bleuler (1968) suggested that the proportion of schizophrenic patients who recover had not significantly increased since the early years of the twentieth century. He observed, however, that the number of "catastrophic" and chronic cases of schizophrenia had decreased, and milder forms of the disease had increased, as a result of the reduction in mishandling and neglect of hospitalized patients that was common earlier in the century. Shepherd et al. (1989) concluded, from their review of twentieth-century outcome studies in schizophrenia, that there had been a substantial improvement in recovery rates since the 1950s. Warner's (1985) more comprehensive review, however, did not confirm this impression: the data indicated that recovery rates had scarcely improved since the early years of the century, though they showed a substantial decline in the 1920s and 1930s.

5

Conclusions and recommendations for future studies

5.1 Methodological issues

Methodological problems, especially lack of standardization of diagnostic criteria, seriously limit the comparability of results reported by different researchers and observed in different societies. In the absence of external validating criteria, schizophrenia remains a clinical concept, and the sampling of cases cannot be guided by anything better than a carefully evaluated knowledge base shared by the greatest possible number of investigators. In this regard, the forthcoming introduction of ICD-10 will represent a step forward in the adoption of uniform, specific diagnostic and descriptive criteria to be used in epidemiological research.

The sample requirements necessary to detect an adequate number of cases in epidemiological research also present methodological difficulties. For schizophrenia—an illness with a relatively low incidence—the multicentre collaborative research approach has advantages over single-centre studies and is more likely to add significantly to epidemiological and clinical knowledge. Large numbers of cases can be accumulated in a relatively short time, and the samples at the different sites allow establishment of robust characteristics of the disorder that are constant across cultures and in populations with different demographic, ecological and biological characteristics.

5.2 High-risk studies

Collaborative studies of people at high risk for schizophrenia could be particularly fruitful. The small samples in the high-risk studies conducted to date and the lack of operationalized diagnostic criteria have been obstacles to achieving significant results. The solution to these problems, together with a focus on promising areas of research, such as attention or information processing markers and smooth-pursuit eye movement, may provide a better understanding of the etiology of schizophrenia (see section 3.6). The ultimate goal of such research would be to find preventive measures or early interventions for those at high risk of developing the disorder (Erlenmeyer-Kimling & Cornblatt, 1987b).

5.3 Geographical stability of incidence

Important new epidemiological data on schizophrenia have been derived from the WHO Study on the Determinants of Outcome of Severe Mental Disorders (Jablensky et al., 1992), which employed a multisite collaborative methodology. The study revealed that incidence rates of schizophrenia, at various levels of definition, are similar across countries: this is especially true for the most restricted definition—the CATEGO S+ class. Even the rates for the most broadly defined diagnostic category (CATEGO S,P,O) varied between centres by a factor of no more than 2.6. The extent to which this degree of variation is seen as important is a matter of perspective. For health administrators, the differences in occurrence of broadly defined schizophrenia may be important for the delivery of health care: for researchers exploring the etiology of the disorders, the similarity of incidence rates at the CATEGO S+ level is an important finding. It is clear, however, that the incidence found in the study was much more stable than earlier research with less standardized diagnostic procedures would have led us to expect.

The absence of marked variation in the incidence of schizophrenia does not lend itself to easy interpretation, in the absence of an understanding of the relationship between the schizophrenic phenotype and the underlying causes and pathophysiology of the disorder. "If schizophrenia is not a single disease of uniform aetiology and pathophysiology, but rather a 'final common pathway' for a variety of pathological processes and developmental anomalies—some with strong genetic contribution and some resulting primarily from environmental factors—then the relatively invariant rate of its occurrence could be the expression of a similarly distributed liability for a schizophrenic type of response to different causes rather than a reflection of a similar distribution of an identical primary cause" (Jablensky, 1989). A "nuclear" schizophrenic syndrome (CATEGO S+ in the Determinants of Outcome study), with its clinical consistency and uniform occurrence, may be a manifestation of a more complex genotype with a much wider range of phenotypical expression.

5.4 Temporal changes in incidence

The issue of whether the incidence of schizophrenia is on the decline or not is a matter of considerable interest and importance. To date, all of the attempts to arrive at an answer to this question have used treatment-related statistics. However, these approaches are unlikely to yield a definitive solution, since the rates are susceptible to variation with changing diagnostic practices and patterns of institutional care. A field survey with a comprehensive sampling strategy is required. For example, it would be productive to repeat the incidence survey of the multisite Determinants of Outcome study ten years or more after drawing the original sample.

5.5 Sex differences

Differences in schizophrenia between males and females may prove to be a productive area of research. The consistent finding of an earlier age of onset among men, together with data showing differences in course and outcome, premorbid functioning, phenomenology, familial risk and brain structure, point to the value of sex differences in establishing subtypes of schizophrenia. "The advantage of using gender as the subdividing variable by which to look for heterogeneity is that it is completely reliable, stable and valid in its definition" (Lewis et al., 1992). It is unlikely, however, that all the sexually dimorphic features of schizophrenia can be explained on the basis of a single model. It will be important in future studies to avoid potential sources of sampling bias that may account for inconsistent findings. Walker & Lewine (1993), for example, have stressed the importance of reporting the sex ratio of the population from which the sample is drawn and the sex ratio of the studied sample.

5.6 Social class and urbanization

Recent data make it clear that social drift alone cannot explain the social-class gradient for schizophrenia or the high prevalence of the disorder in cities (see sections 3.2.7 and 3.2.8). Epidemiological research is required to establish the mediating factors that lead to the greater occurrence of schizophrenia in the lower socioeconomic groups and in urban areas. Besides social drift, such factors may include viral infections, obstetric complications, nutrition, head trauma, stressful life events and work conditions. Link et al. (1986) have shown a relationship between harsh work conditions and the development of schizophrenia in New York City. Similar research to evaluate relationships between the various risk factors and the onset of schizophrenia in rural and urban settings may help to show whether the path to illness is the same in the two types of environment.

5.7 Immigrant status

The observation of increased rates of schizophrenia among Afro-Caribbeans in the United Kingdom and the evidence that the risk for the illness appears substantially greater in second-generation immigrants (see section 3.2.8) raise issues that warrant further investigation. The increased risk in second-generation immigrants may be due to (a) obstetric complications secondary to changes in maternal nutrition, (b) improved fetal survival resulting from better perinatal care, (c) a greater risk of intrauterine or neonatal viral infection, and (d) psychosocial stresses such as family disintegration, homelessness and deprivation (Jablensky, 1993; Warner, 1994). Studies of Afro-Caribbean patients and controls examining obstetric and neonatal history, season of birth, and social factors would yield useful information. Comparative studies in the United Kingdom and the West Indies would reveal whether schizophrenia rates are higher in immigrants than in residents of the country of origin.

5.8 Co-occurring illnesses

The investigation of genetic linkage in schizophrenia may be advanced by studies of illnesses that co-occur with schizophrenia with an increased or decreased incidence. The low rate of occurrence of cancer of the colon and lung in schizophrenic patients (Masterson & O'Shea, 1984; Gulbinat et al., 1992) raises the possibility that a gene that increases the vulnerability to schizophrenia is linked to a cancer-suppressing gene. A large-scale epidemiological survey of cancer risk in schizophrenic patients, their first-degree relatives and the general population could be of considerable interest. A reduced risk for certain carcinomas in the mothers, siblings and children of schizophrenic patients would constitute evidence of a genetic linkage.

5.9 Categorical versus continuous models

Schizophrenia may be conceived of as a distinct syndrome, categorically different from other conditions (the dichotomous/categorical model), or as a vulnerability distributed along a continuum (the continuous/dimensional model). Häfner (1988) observed that most schizophrenic features that appear to be invariable across cultures, such as lack of insight, suspiciousness, delusional mood, ideas of reference, delusions of persecution, and flatness of affect, are dimensional in nature. Further support for the dimensional model comes from psychometric and neurophysiological studies (for example, the reaction-time cross-over phenomenon, retarded modality shift and smooth-pursuit eye movement), in which a distribution along a continuous range of abnormalities is observed.

Häfner (1988) suggested that the model of schizophrenia as a "natural disease entity", as first conceived by Kraepelin in 1896, presents difficulties in interpreting the new epidemiological findings. In searching for the causes of schizophrenia, continuous models, as favoured by Kraepelin in his later years, appear more plausible. Häfner points out that three types of evidence support the continuous model of schizophrenia:

1. the onset of the disorder is often preceded by social and cognitive deficits, by mild schizophrenia-like symptoms, or subclinical speech and thought disorders and emotional instability;
2. in the genetic environment of people with schizophrenia, it is possible to find an increased rate of schizoid, paranoid, and eccentric and odd personalities, and also higher rates of other psychiatric disturbances;
3. the studies that have attempted to identify biological trait variables and vulnerability markers have so far produced unimodal continuous patterns of distribution between schizophrenics and their relatives.

5.10 Social and biological risk factors

Häfner (1990) concluded that "after almost a century of schizophrenia research a strikingly large number of questions on the causes or risk factors specific for premorbid characteristics and on factors determining the onset and course of psychotic episodes and other aspects of the disease, such as social and cognitive deficits, remain unresolved." Genetic factors are clearly important in the development of schizophrenia, but they are not sufficient to explain the entire pattern of occurrence: for example, monozygotic twins are concordant for schizophrenia in only about half of the instances. Neurodevelopmental factors, such as birth injury and maternal infection during gestation, appear to be relevant to the development of the disorder but the influence of these factors has not yet been well defined. Around the world, social class and caste have a complex relationship with the occurrence of schizophrenia, probably reflecting, in different instances, neurodevelopmental effects, social causation and social drift. Social stress, in the form of stressful life events, forms part of the pool of causal factors that affect the onset of the disorder.

The substantially better outcome for schizophrenic patients in developing countries (WHO, 1979; Jablensky et al., 1992) has not yet been satisfactorily explained. Some have argued that the course of the illness is affected by the patterns of utilization of labour in different parts of the world and the greater ease with which a person recovering from a psychotic disorder can return to work in a subsistence economy (Warner, 1985). Although, as some argue, epidemiological knowledge may not support sociocultural models of the *etiology* of schizophrenia (Häfner, 1987), the social environment may be of substantially greater importance in shaping the ultimate course and outcome of the condition. The relationship of the family environment to the course of schizophrenia, for example, has proven to be a productive area of research (Kavanagh, 1992). Further research on the effect of sociocultural variables, especially work, on the course of schizophrenia is clearly needed.

References

Aarachau BM et al. (1972) A checklist for the diagnosis of schizophrenia. *British journal of psychiatry*, 121: 529–539.

Abrams R, Taylor M (1973) First-rank symptoms, severity of illness, and treatment response in schizophrenia. *Comprehensive psychiatry*, 14: 353–355.

Adams W et al. (1993) Epidemiological evidence that maternal influenza contributes to the aetiology of schizophrenia: an analysis of Scottish, English and Danish data. *British journal of psychiatry*, 163: 522–534.

Adelstein AM et al. (1968) The epidemiology of schizophrenia in an English city. *Social psychiatry*, 3: 47–53.

Adler LE et al. (1992) Normalization by nicotine of deficient auditory sensory gating in the relatives of schizophrenics. *Biological psychiatry*, 32: 607–616.

Akimoto H et al. (1943) Chihō shōtoshi ni okeru minseigaku-teki oyobi seishinigaku-teki chosa. *Seishin shinkei gaku zasshi*, 47: 1–24.

Akimoto H et al. (1964) An epidemiological, genetic and social psychiatric study on mental disorders in the isolated island of Hachijo-jima. *Psychiatria et neurologia japonica*, 66: 951–986.

American Psychiatric Association (1980) *Diagnostic and statistical manual of mental disorders*, 3rd ed. Washington, DC, American Psychiatric Press.

American Psychiatric Association (1987) *Diagnostic and statistical manual of mental disorders*, 3rd ed. rev. Washington, DC, American Psychiatric Press.

American Psychiatric Association (1994) *Diagnostic and statistical manual of mental disorders*, 4th ed. Washington, DC, American Psychiatric Press.

Andreasen NC, Flaum M (1991) Schizophrenia: the characteristic symptoms. *Schizophrenia bulletin*, 17: 27–50.

Angermeyer MC, Kuhn L (1988) Gender differences in age at onset of schizophrenia. *European archives of psychiatry and neurological science*, 237: 351–364.

Angst J (1991) Is schizophrenia disappearing? *European archives of psychiatry and clinical neuroscience*, 240: 373–378 (letter).

Anthony JO et al. (1985) Comparison of the lay diagnostic interview schedule and a standardized psychiatric diagnosis: experience in eastern Baltimore. *Archives of general psychiatry*, 42: 667–675.

Arai N et al. (1958) The psychiatric investigation by census in Chichi-bu District and the comparison with another farm village. *Psychiatria et neurologia japonica*, 60: 475–486.

Asarnow JR (1988) Children at risk for schizophrenia: converging lines of evidence. *Schizophrenia bulletin*, 14: 613–631.

Astrachan BM et al. (1972) A checklist for the diagnosis of schizophrenia. *British journal of psychiatry*, 121: 529–536.

Astrup C (1982) *The increase of mental disorders.* Oslo, National Case Register of Mental disorders, Gaustad Hospital (unpublished report).

Averback P (1981) Lesions of the nucleus ansa peduncularis in neuropsychiatric disease. *Archives of neurology*, 38: 230–235.

Baasher T (1961) Survey of mental illness in Wadi Halfa. Paper presented at the Sixth International Congress on Mental Health (cited in Racy J. Psychiatry in the Arab east. *Acta psychiatrica scandinavica*, 1970, 211 (Suppl.): 92–93).

Babigian HM (1980) Schizophrenia: epidemiology. In: Kaplan HI, Freedman AM, Sadock BJ, eds. *Comprehensive textbook of psychiatry*, 3rd ed., vol. 2, Baltimore, Williams & Wilkins, pp. 860–866.

Bamrah JS et al. (1991) Epidemiology in Salford, 1974–84: changes in an urban community over ten years. *British journal of psychiatry*, 159: 802–810.

Barker DJP (1989) Rise and fall of Western diseases. *Nature*, 338: 371–372.

Barker DJP, Phillips DIW (1984) Current incidence of thyrotoxicosis and past prevalence of goitre in 12 British towns. *Lancet*, ii: 567–570.

Barr CE et al. (1990) Exposure to influenza epidemics during gestation and adult schizophrenia: a 40-year study. *Archives of general psychiatry*, 47: 869–874.

Bates CE, van Dam CH (1984) Low incidence of schizophrenia in British Columbia coastal Indians. *Journal of epidemiology and community health*, 38: 127–130.

Bebbington PE (1987) Life events in schizophrenia: the WHO collaborative study. *Social psychiatry*, 22: 179–180.

Beck JC (1978) Social influences on the prognosis of schizophrenia. *Schizophrenia bulletin*, 4: 86–101.

Beiser M, Iacono WG (1990) An update on the epidemiology of schizophrenia. *Canadian journal of psychiatry*, 35: 657–668.

Beiser M et al. (1989) Temporal stability in the major mental disorders. In: Robins LN, Barrett JE, eds. *The validity of psychiatric diagnosis*, New York, Raven Press, pp. 77–97.

Ben-Tovim DI, Cushnie JM (1986) The prevalence of schizophrenia in a remote area of Botswana. *British journal of psychiatry*, 148: 576–580.

Bland RC, Kolada J (1988) Diagnostic issues and current criteria for schizophrenia. In: Tsuang MT, Simpson JC, eds, *Handbook of schizophrenia*. Vol. 3: *Nosology, epidemiology and genetics*. Amsterdam, Elsevier, pp. 1–25.

Bland RC, Parker JH (1978) Prognosis in schizophrenia. *Archives of general psychiatry*, 35: 72–77.

Bland RC et al. (1976) Prognosis in schizophrenia: a ten-year follow-up of first admissions. *Archives of general psychiatry*, 33: 949–954.

Bland RC et al. (1988) Lifetime prevalence of psychiatric disorders in Edmonton. *Acta psychiatrica scandinavica*, 338 (suppl.): 24–32.

Bland RC et al. (1990) Prevalence of psychiatric disorders and suicide attempts in a prison population. *Canadian journal of psychiatry*, 35: 407–413.

Blazer D et al. (1985) Psychiatric disorders. A rural/urban comparison. *Archives of general psychiatry*, 42: 651–656.

Bleuler E (1908) Die Prognose der Dementia Praecox-Schizophreniegruppe. *Allgemeine Zeitschrift für Psychiatrie*, 65: 436–464 (translated and published in: Cutting J, Shepherd M, eds. *The clinical roots of the schizophrenic concept*. Oxford, Oxford University Press, 1987, pp. 59–74).

Bleuler M (1968) A 23-year longitudinal study of 208 schizophrenics and impressions in regard to the nature of schizophrenia. In: Rosenthal D, Kety SS, *The transmission of schizophrenia*, Oxford, Pergamon, p. 3.

Bloom FE (1993) Advancing a neurodevelopmental origin for schizophrenia. *Archives of general psychiatry*, 50: 224–227.

Bojholm S, Stromgren E (1989) Prevalence of schizophrenia on the island of Bornholm in 1935 and in 1983. *Acta psychiatrica scandinavica*, 348 (Suppl.): 157–166.

Böök JA (1953) A genetic and neuropsychiatric investigation of a North-Swedish population. *Acta genetica et statistica medica*, 4: 1–100.

Böök JA et al. (1978) Schizophrenia in a North Swedish geographical isolate, 1900–1977: epidemiology, genetics and biochemistry. *Clinical genetics*, 14: 373–394.

Bowler AE, Torrey EF (1990) Influenza and schizophrenia: Helsinki and Edinburgh. *Archives of general psychiatry*, 47: 876–877 (letter).

Bradbury TN, Miller GA (1985) Season of birth in schizophrenia: a review of evidence, methodology and etiology. *Psychological bulletin*, 98: 569–594.

Breakey WR et al. (1989) Health and mental health problems of homeless men and women in Baltimore. *Journal of the American Medical Association*, 262: 1352–1357.

Bremer J (1951) A social psychiatric investigation of a small community in northern Norway. *Acta psychiatrica et neurologica scandinavica*, 62 (suppl.): 1–166.

Brockington IF et al. (1978) Definitions of schizophrenia: concordance and prediction of outcome. *Psychological medicine*, 8: 387–398.

Bromet E et al. (1988) Basic principles of epidemiologic research in schizophrenia. In: Tsuang MT, Simpson JC, eds, *Handbook of schizophrenia*. Vol. 3: *Nosology, epidemiology and genetics*. Amsterdam, Elsevier, pp.151–168.

Brown GW, Birley JLT (1968) Crises and life changes and the onset of schizophrenia. *Journal of health and social behaviour*, 9: 203–214.

Bruce ML et al. (1991) Poverty and psychiatric status. *Archives of general psychiatry*, 48: 470–474.

Brugger C (1931) Versuch einer Geisteskrankenzählung in Thüringen. *Zeitschrift für die gesamte Neurologie und Psychiatrie*, 133: 252–290.

Brugger C (1933) Psychiatrische Ergebnisse einer medizinischen, anthropologischen und soziologischen Bevölkerungsuntersuchung. *Zeitschrift für die gesamte Neurologie und Psychiatrie*, 146: 489–524.

Brugger C (1938) Psychiatrische Bestandesaufnahme im Gebiet eines medizinisch-änthropologischen Zensus in der Nähe von Rosenheim. *Zeitschrift für die gesamte Neurologie und Psychiatrie*, 160: 189–207.

Burnam MA et al. (1987) Six month prevalence of specific psychiatric disorders among Mexican Americans and non-Hispanic whites in Los Angeles. *Archives of general psychiatry*, 44: 687–694.

Cabot MR (1990) The incidence and prevalence of schizophrenia in the Republic of Ireland. *Social psychiatry and psychiatric epidemiology*, 25: 210–215.

Cade JFJ, Krupinski J (1962) Incidence of psychiatric disorders in Victoria in relation to country of birth. *Medical journal of Australia*, 49: 400–404.

Canino GJ et al. (1987) The prevalence of specific psychiatric disorders in Puerto Rico. *Archives of general psychiatry*, 44: 727–735.

Carpenter WT, Buchanan RW (1994) Schizophrenia. *New England journal of medicine*, 330: 681–690.

Carpenter WT Jr, Strauss JS (1973) Are there pathognomonic symptoms in schizophrenia? An empirical investigation of Schneider's first-rank symptoms. *Archives of general psychiatry*, 28: 847–852.

Carpenter WT Jr, Strauss JS (1974) Cross-cultural evaluation of Schneider's first rank symptoms of schizophrenia: a report from the international pilot study of schizophrenia. *American journal of psychiatry*, 131: 682–687.

Carstairs GM, Kapur RL (1976) *The great universe of Kota: a study of stress, change, and mental disorder in an Indian village*. Berkeley, University of California Press.

Casey PR et al. (1984) The diagnostic status of patients with conspicuous psychiatric morbidity in primary care. *Psychological medicine*, 14: 673–681.

Castle DJ (1993) Some current controversies in the epidemiology of schizophrenia. *Current medical literature, psychiatry*, 4 (1): 3–7.

Castle D et al. (1991) The incidence of operationally defined schizophrenia in Camberwell, 1965–84. *British journal of psychiatry*, 159: 790–794.

Chandrasena R (1987) Schneider's first rank symptoms: an international and inter-ethnic comparative study. *Acta psychiatrica scandinavica*, 76: 574–578.

Cheung P (1991) Adult psychiatric epidemiology in China in the 80s. *Culture, medicine and psychiatry*, 15: 479–496.

Clark RE (1949) Psychoses, income and occupational prestige. *American journal of sociology*, 54: 433–440.

Cochrane R (1977) Mental illness in immigrants to England and Wales: an analysis of mental hospital admissions, 1971. *Social psychiatry*, 12: 25–35.

Cochrane R, Bal SS (1987) Migration and schizophrenia: an examination of five hypotheses. *Social psychiatry*, 22: 181–191.

Cochrane R, Bal SS (1988) Ethnic density is unrelated to incidence of schizophrenia. *British journal of psychiatry*, 153: 363–366.

Coid J (1984) How many psychiatric patients in prison? *British journal of psychiatry*, 145: 78–86.

Cooper JE et al. (1972) *Psychiatric diagnosis in New York and London*. London, Oxford University Press (Maudsley Monograph No. 20).

Cooper JE et al. (1987) The incidence of schizophrenia in Nottingham. *British journal of psychiatry*, 151: 619–626.

Copeland JRM et al. (1991) The epidemiology of dementia. GMS-AGESCAT studies of prevalence and incidence, including studies in progress. *European archives of psychiatry and neurological science*, 240: 212–217.

Crocetti GM et al. (1971) Selected aspects of the epidemiology of psychoses in Croatia, Yugoslavia. III. The cluster sample and the results of the pilot survey. *American journal of epidemiology*, 94: 126–134.

Crow TJ (1980) Molecular pathology of schizophrenia: more than one disease process? *British medical journal*, 280: 66–68.

Crow TJ (1990) Trends in schizophrenia. *Lancet*, 335: 851 (letter).

Crow TJ, Done DJ (1992) Prenatal exposure to influenza does not cause schizophrenia. *British journal of psychiatry*, 161: 390–393.

Curran JP, Cirelli VA (1988) The role of psychosocial factors in the etiology, course and outcome of schizophrenia. In: Tsuang MT, Simpson JC, eds. *Handbook of schizophrenia. Vol. 3: Nosology, epidemiology and genetics.* Amsterdam, Elsevier, pp. 275–297.

Dahl AA et al. (1992) Convergence of American and Scandinavian diagnoses of functional psychoses. *Comprehensive psychiatry*, 33: 13–16.

Dalén P (1968) Month of birth and schizophrenia. *Acta psychiatrica scandinavica*, 203: 55–60.

Dalén P (1975) *Season of birth: a study of schizophrenia and other mental disorders.* Amsterdam, North Holland.

Dalén P (1990) Deviant birth season distribution: does it offer a clue to the aetiology of schizophrenia? In: Häfner H, Gattaz WF, eds. *Search for the causes of schizophrenia*, Vol 2. Berlin, Springer-Verlag, pp. 7–13.

Day R et al.(1987) Stressful life events preceding the acute onset of schizophrenia: a cross-national study from the World Health Organization. *Culture, medicine and psychiatry*, 11: 123–205.

de Alarcon J et al. (1990) Trends in schizophrenia. *Lancet*, 335: 852–853 (letter).

de Sauvage NWJJ (1934) Verband tussen geboortemaand en schizophrene en manisch-depressieve geesteszieken. *Nederlandsch tijdschrift voor geneeskunde*, 79: 528.

de Sauvage NWJJ (1951) Verband tussen geboortemaand en schizophrene en manisch-depressieve geesteszieken. *Nederlandsch tijdschrift voor geneeskunde*, 4: 3855–3864.

de Sauvage NWJJ (1954) Vitamin C and the schizophrenic syndrome. *Folia psychiatrica, neurologica et neurochirurgica Neerlandica*, 57: 347–355.

Der G et al. (1990) Is schizophrenia disappearing? *Lancet*, 335: 513–516.

Dickson WE, Kendell RE (1986) Does maintenance lithium therapy prevent recurrences of mania under ordinary clinical conditions? *Psychological medicine*, 16: 521–530.

Dilling H (1980) Psychiatric and primary health services: results of a field study. *Acta psychiatrica scandinavica*, 285 (Suppl.):15–22.

Dilling H, Weyerer S (1980) Incidence and prevalence of treated mental disorders; health care planning in a small town region of Upper Bavaria. *Acta psychiatrica scandinavica*, 61: 209–222.

Dilling H, Weyerer S (1984) Prevalence of mental disorders in the small-town, rural region of Traunstein (Upper Bavaria). *Acta psychiatrica scandinavica*, 69: 60–79.

Dilling H et al. (1989) The Upper Bavarian studies. *Acta psychiatrica scandinavica*, 348 (Suppl.): 113–140.

Dohrenwend BP et al. (1987) Social and psychological risk factors for episodes of schizophrenia. In: Häfner H et al., eds. *Search for the causes of schizophrenia*, Berlin, Springer-Verlag, pp. 275–296.

Dohrenwend BP et al. (1992) Socioeconomic status and psychiatric disorders: the causation-selection issue. *Science*, 255: 946–952.

Done DJ et al. (1991) Complications of pregnancy and delivery in relation to psychosis in adult life: data from the British perinatal mortality survey sample. *British medical journal*, 302: 1576–1580.

Dube KC, Kumar N (1972) Epidemiological study of schizophrenia. *Journal of biosocial science*, 4: 187–195.

Dunham HW (1965) *Community and schizophrenia: an epidemiological analysis.* Detroit, Wayne State University Press.

Eagles JM (1991a) Is schizophrenia disappearing? *British journal of psychiatry*, 158: 834–835.

Eagles JM (1991b) The relationship between schizophrenia and immigration: are there alternatives to psychosocial models? *British journal of psychiatry*, 159: 783–789.

Eagles JM, Whalley LJ (1985) Decline in the diagnosis of schizophrenia among first admissions to Scottish mental hospitals from 1969–78. *British journal of psychiatry*, 146: 151–154.

Eagles JM et al. (1988) Decline in the diagnosis of schizophrenia among first contacts with psychiatric services in north-east Scotland, 1969–1984. *British journal of psychiatry*, 152: 793–798.

Eagles JM et al. (1990) Obstetric complications in DSM-III schizophrenics and their siblings. *Lancet*, 335: 1139–1141.

Eastwell H (1975) Schizophrenic typology in Aboriginal Australia: observations from Arnhem Land (unpublished paper cited in Torrey EF, *Schizophrenia and civilization*, New York, Jason Aronson, pp. 144–145).

Eaton JW, Weil RJ (1955) *Culture and mental disorders.* Glencoe, Free Press.

Eaton WW (1974) Residence, social class, and schizophrenia. *Journal of health and social behavior*, 15: 289–299.

Eaton WW (1975) Marital status and schizophrenia. *Acta psychiatrica scandinavica*, 52: 320–329.

Eaton WW (1985) Epidemiology of schizophrenia. *Epidemiological reviews*, 7: 105–126.

Eaton WW (1991) Update on the epidemiology of schizophrenia. *Epidemiologic reviews*, 13: 320–328.

Eaton WW et al. (1988) The use of epidemiology for risk factor research in schizophrenia: an overview and methodologic critique. In: Tsuang MT, Simpson JC, eds. *Handbook of schizophrenia. Vol. 3: Nosology, epidemiology and genetics.* Amsterdam, Elsevier, pp. 169–204.

Eaton WW et al. (1991) Screening for psychosis in the general population with a self-report interview. *Journal of nervous and mental disease,* 179: 689–693.

Eaton WW et al. (1992a) Schizophrenia and rheumatoid arthritis: a review. *Schizophrenia research,* 6: 181–192.

Eaton WW et al. (1992b) Long-term course of hospitalization for schizophrenia. Part I. Risk for rehospitalization. *Schizophrenia bulletin,* 18: 217–228.

Egeland JA, Hostetter AM (1983) Amish study. I: Affective disorders among the Amish, 1976–1980. *American journal of psychiatry,* 140: 56–61.

Ellard J (1987) Did schizophrenia exist before the eighteenth century? *Australia and New Zealand journal of psychiatry,* 21: 306–314.

Elnagar MN et al. (1971) Mental health in an Indian rural community. *British journal of psychiatry,* 118: 499–503.

Endicott JN et al. (1982) Diagnostic criteria for schizophrenia. *Archives of general psychiatry,* 39: 884–889.

Erlenmeyer-Kimling L, Cornblatt B (1987a) The New York High-Risk Project: a follow-up report. *Schizophrenia bulletin,* 13: 451–461.

Erlenmeyer-Kimling L, Cornblatt B (1987b) High-risk research in schizophrenia: a summary of what has been learned. *Journal of psychiatric research,* 4: 401–411.

Essen-Moller E (1956) Individual traits and morbidity in a Swedish rural population. *Acta psychiatrica et neurologica scandinavica,* 100 (Suppl.): 1–160.

Fananas L et al. (1989) Seasonality of birth in schizophrenia: an insufficient stratification of control population. *Social psychiatry and psychiatric epidemiology,* 24: 266–270.

Faraone SV et al. (1994) Gender differences in age at onset of schizophrenia. *British journal of psychiatry,* 164: 625–629.

Faris REL, Dunham HW (1939) *Mental disorders in urban areas: an ecological study of schizophrenia and other psychoses.* Chicago, University of Chicago Press.

Feighner JP et al. (1972) Diagnostic criteria for use in psychiatric research. *Archives of general psychiatry,* 26: 57–63.

Fenton WS et al. (1981) Diagnosis of schizophrenia: a critical review of current diagnostic systems. *Schizophrenia bulletin,* 7: 452–476.

Fischer PJ, Breakey WR (1991) The epidemiology of alcohol, drug, and mental disorders among homeless persons. *American psychologist,* 46: 1115–1128.

Folnegović Z et al. (1990) The incidence of schizophrenia in Croatia. *British journal of psychiatry*, 156: 363–365.

Folnegović Z, Folnegović-Šmalc V (1992) Schizophrenia in Croatia: interregional differences in prevalence and a comment on constant incidence. *Journal of epidemiology and community health*, 46: 248–255.

Franzen G, Ingvar DH (1975) Abnormal distribution of cerebral activity in chronic schizophrenia. *Journal of psychiatric research*, 12: 199–214.

Freedman R et al. (1991) Elementary neuronal dysfunctions in schizophrenia. *Schizophrenia research*, 4: 233–243.

Freeman H, Alpert M (1986) Prevalence of schizophrenia in an urban population. *British journal of psychiatry*, 149: 603–611.

Fremming KH (1951) *The expectations of mental infirmity in a sample of the Danish population*. London, Cassell.

Fugelli P (1975) Mental health and living conditions in a fishing community in northern Norway. *Acta psychiatrica scandinavica*, 263 (Suppl.): 39–42.

Gardner EA, Babigian HM (1966) A longitudinal comparison of psychiatric service to selected socioeconomic areas of Monroe County (New York). *American journal of orthopsychiatry*, 36: 818–828.

Geddes JR et al. (1993) Persistence of the decline in the diagnosis of schizophrenia among first admissions to Scottish hospitals from 1969 to 1988. *British journal of psychiatry*, 163: 620–626.

Geddes J et al. (1994) Comparison of prevalence of schizophrenia among residents of hostels for homeless people in 1966 and 1992. *British medical journal*, 308: 816–819.

Gerard DL, Houston LG (1953) Family setting and the social ecology of schizophrenia. *Psychiatric quarterly*, 27: 90–101.

Giel DR et al (1980) Over de epidemiologie van functionele psychosen en invaliditeit. *Tijdschrift voor psychiatrie*, 22: 710–722.

Giggs JA, Cooper JE (1987) Ecological structure and the distribution of schizophrenia and affective psychoses in Nottingham. *British journal of psychiatry*, 151: 627–633.

Glatzel J (1990) Psychiatric diagnosis in the German-speaking countries. In: Sartorius N et al., eds. *Sources and traditions of classification in psychiatry*. Bern, Hogrefe & Huber, pp. 58–92.

Goldberg EM, Morrison SL (1963) Schizophrenia and social class. *British journal of psychiatry*, 109: 785–802.

Goodman R (1988) Are complications of pregnancy and birth causes of schizophrenia? *Developmental medicine and child neurology*, 30: 391–395.

Gottesman II (1991) *Schizophrenia genesis: the origins of madness.* New York, Freeman.

Gottesman II, Shields J (1982) *Schizophrenia: the epigenetic puzzle.* New York, Cambridge University Press.

Graham PM (1990) Trends in schizophrenia. *Lancet*, 335: 1214 (letter).

Griffiths R et al. (1989) Ethnic differences in birth statistics from central Birmingham. *British medical journal*, 298: 94–95.

Gulbinat W et al. (1992) Cancer incidence of schizophrenic patients: results of record linkage studies in three countries. *British journal of psychiatry*, 161 (Suppl. 18): 75–85.

Gunderson JG, Mosher LR (1975) The cost of schizophrenia. *American journal of psychiatry*, 132: 901–6.

Gunn J et al. (1978) *Psychiatric aspects of imprisonment.* London, Academic Press.

Gunn J et al. (1991) Treatment needs of prisoners with psychiatric disorders. *British medical journal*, 303: 338–341.

Gupta S (1993) Can environmental factors explain the epidemiology of schizophrenia in immigrant groups? *Social psychiatry and psychiatric epidemiology*, 28: 263–266.

Gupta S, Murray RM (1991) The changing incidence of schizophrenia: fact or artefact? *Directions in psychiatry*, 11: 1–8.

Häfner H (1987) Epidemiology of schizophrenia. In: Häfner H et al., eds. *Search for the causes of schizophrenia.* Vol. I. Berlin, Springer-Verlag, pp. 47–74.

Häfner H (1988) What is schizophrenia? Changing perspectives in epidemiology. *European archives of psychiatry and neurological sciences*, 238: 63–72.

Häfner H (1989) Application of epidemiological research toward a model for the etiology of schizophrenia. *Schizophrenia research*, 2: 375–383.

Häfner H (1990) New perspectives in the epidemiology of schizophrenia. In: Häfner H, Gattaz WF, eds. *Search for the causes of schizophrenia,* Vol II. Berlin, Springer-Verlag, pp. 408–431.

Häfner H, an der Heiden W (1986) The Mannheim case register: the long-stay population. In: ten Horn GHMM et al., eds. *Psychiatric case registers in public health.* Amsterdam, Elsevier, pp. 28–38.

Häfner H, Gattaz WF (1991) Is schizophrenia disappearing? *European archives of psychiatry and clinical neuroscience*, 240: 374–376.

Häfner H, Reimann H (1970) Spatial distribution of mental disorders in Mannheim, 1965. In: Hare EH, Wing JK, eds. *Psychiatric epidemiology,* London, Oxford University Press, pp. 341–354.

Häfner H et al. (1987) Abnormal seasonality of schizophrenic births: a specific finding? *European archives of psychiatry and neurological sciences*, 236: 333–342.

Häfner H et al. (1989) How does gender influence age at first hospitalization for schizophrenia? *Psychological medicine*, 19: 903–918.

Häfner H et al. (1991a) An animal model for the effects of estradiol on dopamine-mediated behavior: implications for sex differences in schizophrenia. *Psychiatry research*, 38: 125–134.

Häfner H et al. (1991b) Oestradiol enhances the vulnerability threshold for schizophrenia in women by an early effect on dopaminergic neurotransmission. Evidence from an epidemiological study and from animal experiments. *European archives of psychiatry and clinical neuroscience*, 241: 65–68.

Häfner H et al. (1992). First onset and early symptomatology of schizophrenia. A chapter of epidemiological and neurobiological research into age and sex differences. *European archives of psychiatry and clinical neuroscience*, 242: 109–118.

Häfner H et al. (1993). The influence of age and sex on the onset and early course in schizophrenia. *British journal of psychiatry*, 162: 80–86.

Hagnell O (1966) *A prospective study of the incidence of mental disorder*. Lund, Norstedts-Bonniers.

Hagnell O et al. (1990) *The incidence of mental illness over a quarter of a century: the Lundby longitudinal study of mental illnesses in a total population based on 42,000 observation years*. Stockholm, Almquist & Wiksell International.

Hailey AM et al. (1974) *Psychiatric services in Camberwell and Salford: statistics from the Camberwell and Salford Registers: 1964–1973*. London, MRC Social Psychiatry Unit.

Halevi HS (1963) Frequency of mental illness among Jews in Israel. *International journal of social psychiatry*, 9: 268–282.

Halldin T (1984) Prevalence of mental disorder in an urban population in central Sweden. *Acta psychiatrica scandinavica*, 69: 503–518.

Hambrecht M et al. (1992) Gender differences in schizophrenia in three cultures. Results of the WHO collaborative study on psychiatric disability. *Social psychiatry and psychiatric epidemiology*, 27: 117–121.

Hambrecht M et al. (1992) Evidence for a gender bias in epidemiological studies of schizophrenia. *Schizophrenia research*, 8: 223–231.

Hambrecht M et al. (1994) Higher mortality risk for schizophrenia in males: fact or fiction? *Comprehensive psychiatry*, 35: 39–49.

Harding TW et al. (1980) Mental disorders in primary care: a study of their frequency and diagnosis in four developing countries. *Psychological medicine*, 10: 231–241.

Hare EH (1956) Mental illness and social conditions in Bristol. *Journal of mental science*, 102: 349–357.

Hare EH (1983) Was insanity on the increase? *British journal of psychiatry*, 142: 439–445.

91

Hare EH (1986) Aspects of the epidemiology of schizophrenia. *British journal of psychiatry*, 149: 554–561.

Hare EH (1987) Epidemiology of schizophrenia and affective psychoses. *British medical bulletin*, 43: 514–530.

Hare EH (1988a) Temporal factors and trends, including birth seasonality and the viral hypothesis. In: Tsuang MT, Simpson JC, eds. *Handbook of schizophrenia. Vol. 3: Nosology, epidemiology and genetics*. Amsterdam, Elsevier, pp. 345–377.

Hare EH (1988b) Schizophrenia as a recent disease. *British journal of psychiatry*, 153: 521–531.

Hare EH, Moran P (1981) A relation between seasonal temperature and the birth rate of schizophrenic patients. *Acta psychiatrica scandinavica*, 63: 396–405.

Hare EH, Price JS (1968) Mental disorder and season of birth: comparison of psychoses with neuroses. *British journal of psychiatry*, 115: 533–540.

Hare EH et al. (1974) Mental disorder and season of birth: a national sample compared with the general population. *British journal of psychiatry*, 124: 81–86.

 Harrison G, Mason P (1993) Schizophrenia—falling incidence and better outcome? *British journal of psychiatry*, 163: 535–541.

Harrison G et al. (1988) A prospective study of severe mental disorder in Afro-Caribbean patients. *Psychological medicine*, 18: 643–657.

Harrison G et al. (1991) Changes in the administrative incidence of schizophrenia. *British journal of psychiatry*, 159: 811–816.

Haruki S (1972) A psychiatric, epidemiological, and socio-psychiatric survey on mental disorders in Tsuma-mura, Okinoshima Island, Shimane Prefecture. *Psychiatria et neurologia japonica*, 71: 301–311.

Helgason T (1964) Epidemiology of mental disorders in Iceland. *Acta psychiatrica scandinavica*, (Suppl.): 173.

Helgason L (1977) Psychiatric services and mental illness in Iceland. *Acta psychiatrica scandinavica*, (Suppl.): 258.

Helzer JE (1988) Uses of structured diagnostic interviews for clinical practice and research in schizophrenia. In: Tsuang MT, Simpson JC, eds. *Handbook of schizophrenia. Vol. 3: Nosology, epidemiology and genetics*. Amsterdam, Elsevier, pp. 41–61.

Helzer JE et al. (1981) Renard diagnostic interview. *Archives of general psychiatry*, 38: 393–398.

Helzer JE et al. (1985) A comparison of clinical and DIS diagnoses: physician reexamination of lay interviewed cases in the general population. *Archives of general psychiatry*, 42: 657–666.

Henderson AS, Burrow GD (1988) *Handbook of social psychiatry*. Amsterdam, Elsevier.

Heston LL (1966) Psychiatric disorders in foster home reared children of schizophrenic mothers. *British journal of psychiatry*, 112: 819–825.

Hiratsuka T, Nomura A (1941) A psychiatric investigation by census in a village, Kanagawa Prefecture. *Japanese journal of health and human ecology*, 9: 436–455.

Hirayasu T (1969) An epidemiological and sociopsychiatric study on the mental and neurological disorders in an isolated island in Okinawa. *Psychiatria et neurologia japonica*, 71: 466–491.

Hollingshead AB, Redlich FC (1958) *Social class and mental illness*. New York, Wiley.

Holzer CE et al. (1986) The increased risk for specific psychiatric disorders among persons of low socioeconomic status. *American journal of social psychiatry*, 4: 259–271.

Hwu HG et al. (1989) Prevalence of psychiatric disorders in Taiwan defined by the Chinese diagnostic interview schedule. *Acta psychiatrica scandinavica*, 79: 136–147.

Iacono WG, Beiser M (1992) Are males more likely than females to develop schizophrenia? *American journal of psychiatry*, 149: 1070–1074.

Jablensky A (1986) Epidemiology of schizophrenia: a European perspective. *Schizophrenia bulletin*, 12: 52–73.

Jablensky A (1988) Schizophrenia and the environment. In: Henderson S, Burrows G, eds. *Handbook of social psychiatry*. Amsterdam, Elsevier, pp. 103–116.

Jablensky A (1989) An overview of the World Health Organization multicentre studies of schizophrenia. In: Williams P et al., eds. *The scope of epidemiological psychiatry: essays in honour of Micheal Shepherd*. London, Routledge, pp. 455–471.

Jablensky A (1993) The epidemiology of schizophrenia. *Current opinion in psychiatry*, 6: 43–52.

Jablensky A, Sartorius N (1975) Culture and schizophrenia. *Psychological medicine*, 5: 113–124.

Jablensky A, Sartorius N (1987) Is schizophrenia universal? *Acta psychiatrica Scandinavica*, 344 (Suppl.): 65–70.

Jablensky A et al. (1987) Incidence worldwide of schizophrenia. *British journal of psychiatry*, 151: 408–421 (letter).

Jablensky A et al. (1992) Schizophrenia: manifestations, incidence and course in different cultures. A World Health Organization ten-country study. *Psychological medicine*, Suppl. 20.

Jaco EG (1960) *Social epidemiology of mental disorders: a psychiatric survey of Texas*. New York, Russell Sage Foundation.

Jacobsen B, Kinney DK (1980) Perinatal complications in adopted and non-adopted schizophrenics and their controls: preliminary results. *Acta psychiatrica scandinavica*, 285 (Suppl.): 337–346.

Japanese Ministry of Health and Welfare (1955) *Nationwide prevalence survey of mental disorders in 1954, Tokyo,* (unpublished mimeograph cited in: Kato M (1969) Psychiatric epidemiological surveys in Japan: the problem of case finding. In: Caudill M, Lin T, eds. *Mental health research in Asia and the Pacific.* Honolulu, East–West Center Press, pp. 92–104).

Japanese Ministry of Health and Welfare (1965) Wagakuni ni okerv seishin-shōgai no genjō. Tokyo: Kōsei-shōshū Eisei Kyoku (cited in Kato M (1969) Psychiatric epidemiological surveys in Japan: the problem of case finding. In: Caudill M, Lin T, eds. *Mental health research in Asia and the Pacific.* Honolulu, East–West Center Press, pp. 92–104).

Jayasundera MG (1969) Mental health surveys in Ceylon. In: Caudill M, Lin T, eds. *Mental health research in Asia and the Pacific.* Honolulu, East–West Center Press, pp. 54–65.

Jeste DV et al. (1985) Did schizophrenia exist before the eighteenth century? *Comprehensive psychiatry,* 26: 493–503.

Jones IH, Horne DJ de L (!973) Psychiatric disorders among Aborigines of the Australian Western Desert: further data and discussion. *Social science and medicine,* 7: 219–228.

Jones PB et al. (1993) Premorbid social underachievement in schizophrenia: results from the Camberwell Collaborative Study. *British journal of psychiatry,* 162: 65–71.

Joyce PR (1987) Changing trends in first admissions and readmissions for mania and schizophrenia in New Zealand. *Australian and New Zealand journal of psychiatry,* 21: 82–86.

Kaila M (1942) Über die Durchschnittschäufigkeit der Geisteskrankheiten und des Schwachsinns in Finland. *Acta psychiatrica et neurologica scandinavica,* 17: 47–67.

Kaličanin P (1987) *Primena epidemioľskog metoda psihijatriji-epidemiološki aspekti schizofrenije u Beogradu.* Belgrade, Institut za stručno usavršavanje i specijalizaciju zdravstvenih radnika.

Kato M (1969) Psychiatric epidemiological surveys in Japan: the problem of case finding. In: Caudill M, Lin T, eds. *Mental health research in Asia and the Pacific.* Honolulu, East–West Center Press, pp. 92–104.

Kavanagh DJ (1992) Recent developments in expressed emotion and schizophrenia. *British journal of psychiatry,* 160: 601–620.

Keith SJ et al. (1991) Schizophrenic disorders in America. In: Robins L, Regier DA, eds. *Psychiatric disorders in America.* New York, Free Press, pp. 33–51.

Kendell RE (1987) Diagnosis and classification of functional psychoses. *British medical bulletin,* 43: 499–513.

Kendell RE, Adams W (1991) Unexplained fluctuations in the risk of schizophrenia by month and year of birth. *British journal of psychiatry,* 158: 758–763.

Kendell RE, Kemp IW (1987) Winter-born v summer-born schizophrenics. *British journal of psychiatry*, 151: 499–505.

Kendell RE, Kemp IW (1989) Maternal influenza in the etiology of schizophrenia. *Archives of general psychiatry*, 46: 878–882.

Kendell RE et al. (1979) Prognostic implications of six alternative definitions of schizophrenia. *Archives of general psychiatry*, 35: 25–31.

Kendell RE et al. (1993) The problem of detecting changes in the incidence of schizophrenia. *British journal of psychiatry*, 162: 212–218.

Kendler K (1990) Familial risk factors and the familial aggregation of psychiatric disorders. *Psychological medicine*, 20: 311–319.

Kendler KS et al. (1989) Psychotic disorders in DSM-III-R. *American journal of psychiatry*, 146: 953–963.

Kendrick T et al. (1991) Role of general practitioners in care of long term mentally ill patients. *British medical journal*, 302: 508–510.

Kessler RC et al. (1987) Psychiatric diagnoses of medical service users: evidence from the epidemiologic catchment area program. *American journal of public health*, 77: 18–23.

Kessler RC et al. (1994) Lifetime and 12-month prevalence of DSM-III-R psychiatric disorders in the United States. *Archives of general psychiatry*, 51: 8–19.

Kety SS (1988) Schizophrenic illness in the families of schizophrenic adoptees: findings from the Danish national sample. *Schizophrenia bulletin*, 14: 217–222.

Khandelwal SK, Workneh F (1988) Psychiatric outpatients in a general hospital in Ethiopia: diagnostic and sociodemographic characteristics. *International journal of social psychiatry*, 34: 230–235.

Klee GD et al. (1967) An ecological analysis of diagnosed mental illness in Baltimore. In: Monroe RR et al., eds. *Psychiatric epidemiology and mental health planning*, Washington, DC, American Psychiatric Association, pp. 107–148.

Klemperer J (1933) Zur Belastungsstatistik der Durchschnitts bevölkerung. Psychose-häufigkeit unter 1000 stichprobemässig ausgelesenen Probanden. *Zeitschrift für die gesamte Neurologie und Psychiatrie*, 146: 277–316.

Koegel P et al. (1988) The prevalence of specific psychiatric disorders among homeless individuals in the inner city of Los Angeles. *Archives of general psychiatry*, 45: 1085–1092.

Koehler K et al. (1977) First-rank symptoms of schizophrenia in Schneider-oriented German centers. *Archives of general psychiatry*, 34: 810–813.

Kohn ML (1973) Social class and schizophrenia: a critical review and a reformulation. *Schizophrenia bulletin*, 7: 60–79.

Kraepelin E (1896) Dementia praecox. In: *Psychiatrie. 5th ed.* Leipzig, Barth. Translated and published in: Cutting J, Shepherd M, eds. (1987), *The clinical roots of the schizophrenic concept.* Oxford, Oxford University Press, pp. 13–24.

Kraepelin E (1909) *Psychiatrie.* 9th ed. Leipzig, Barth.

Kraepelin E (1926) General paralysis. *Journal of nervous and mental disease*, 63: 209–218.

Kraepelin E (1927) *Dementia praecox and paraphrenia.* Edinburgh, Livingstone.

Kramer K (1969) Cross-national study of diagnosis of the mental disorders: origin of the problem. *American journal of psychiatry*, 125 (Suppl.): 1–11.

Kramer M (1957) Discussion of the context of prevalence and incidence as related to epidemiologic studies of mental disorders. *American journal of public health*, 48: 826.

Kramer M (1978) Population changes and schizophrenia, 1970–1985. In: Wynne LC et al., eds. *The nature of schizophrenia: new approaches to research and treatment.* New York, Wiley, pp. 545–571.

Kramer M et al. (1961) Studies of the incidence and prevalence of hospitalized mental disorders in the United Staes: current status and future goals. In: Hoch PH, Lubin J, eds. *Comparative epidemiology of the mental disorders*, New York, Grune & Stratton, pp. 56–100.

Krasik ED, Semin IR (1980) Epidemiological aspects of first admissions of schizophrenic patients. *Zhurnal nevropatologij psikijatrii*, 80: 1354–1359.

Krupinski J (1983) *Admissions, discharges and deaths, 1979–1980.* Melbourne, Mental Health Research Institute, Health Commission of Victoria (Statistical Bulletin No. 15).

Krupinski J, Alexander L (1983) Patterns of psychiatric morbidity in Victoria, Australia, in relation to changes in diagnostic criteria 1948–1978. *Social psychiatry*, 18: 61–67.

Kulcar Z et al. (1971) Selected aspects of the epidemiology of psychoses in Croatia, Yugoslavia: pilot study of communities. *American journal of epidemiology*, 94: 118–125.

Kuriansky JB et al. (1974) On trends in the diagnosis of schizophrenia. *American journal of psychiatry*, 131: 402–408.

Lamb HR, Grant RW (1982) The mentally ill in an urban county jail. *Archives of general psychiatry*, 39: 17–22.

Lane E, Albee GW (1966) Comparative birthweights of schizophrenics and their siblings. *Journal of psychiatry*, 64: 227–231.

Larsson T, Sjögren T (1954) A methodological, psychiatric, and statistical study of a large Swedish rural population. *Acta psychiatrica et neurologica scandinavica*, (Suppl.): 89.

Lee CK et al. (1990a) Psychiatric epidemiology in Korea. Part I: Gender and age differences in Seoul. *Journal of nervous and mental disease*, 178: 242–246.

Lee CK et al. (1990b) Psychiatric epidemiology in Korea. Part II: Urban and rural differences. *Journal of nervous and mental disease*, 178: 247–252.

Leff J (1988) *Psychiatry around the globe: a transcultural view*, 2nd ed. London, Gaskell.

Lehtinen V et al. (1978) Preventive implications of a social-psychiatric survey in the Finnish population. *Psychiatria fennica*, 78: 143–151.

Lehtinen V et al. (1990a) Prevalence of mental disorders among adults in Finland: basic results from the Mini Finland Health Survey. *Acta psychiatrica scandinavica*, 81: 418–425.

Lehtinen V et al. (1990b) The prevalence of PSE-CATEGO disorders in a Finnish adult population cohort. *Social psychiatry and psychiatric epidemiology*, 25: 187–192.

Leighton DC et al. (1963) *The character of danger: the Stirling County study of psychiatric disorder and sociocultural environment. Volume III. Psychiatric symptoms in selected communities*. New York, Basic Books.

Lemkau PV et al. (1942) Mental hygiene problems in an urban district. *Mental hygiene*, 25: 624–646.

Lemkau PV et al. (1943) Mental hygiene problems in an urban district: second paper. *Mental hygiene*, 26: 100–119.

Levav I et al. (1989) Salud mental para todos en America Latina y el Caribe. Bases epidemiologicas para el acción. *Boletino de la Oficina Sanitaria Panamericana*, 107: 196–219.

Lewine RRJ (1981) Sex differences in schizophrenia: timing or subtypes? *Psychological bulletin*, 90: 432–444.

Lewis G et al. (1992) Schizophrenia and city life. *Lancet*, 340: 137–140.

Lewis MS (1989) Age incidence and schizophrenia. Part 1. The season of birth controversy. *Schizophrenia bulletin*, 15: 59–73.

Lewis S (1992) Sex and schizophrenia: vive la différence. *British journal of psychiatry*, 161: 445–450.

Lewis SW, Murray RM (1987) Obstetric complications, neurodevelopmental deviance and risk of schizophrenia. *Journal of psychiatric research*, 21: 413–421.

Liebermann YI (1974) On the problem of incidence of schizophrenia: materials from a clinical and epidemiological survey. *Zhurnal nevropatologii psikijatrii*, 74: 1224–1231.

Lin KM et al. (1981) Overview of mental disorders in Chinese cultures: review of epidemiological and clinical studies. In: Kleinman A, Lin TY, eds. *Normal and abnormal behaviour in Chinese cultures*. Dordrecht, Reidel, pp. 237–272.

Lin T (1953) A study of the incidence of mental disorder in Chinese and other cultures. *Psychiatry*, 16: 313–336.

Lin T et al. (1969) Mental disorders in Taiwan, fifteen years later: a preliminary report. In: Caudill M, Lin T, eds. *Mental health research in Asia and the Pacific*. Honolulu, East–West Center Press, pp. 66–91.

Lin TY et al. (1989) Effects of social change on mental disorders in Taiwan: observations based on a 15-year follow-up survey of general populations in three communities. *Acta psychiatrica scandinavica*, 79 (Suppl. 348): 11–34.

Link B, Dohrenwend BP (1980) Formulation of hypotheses about the ratio of untreated to treated cases in the true prevalence studies of functional psychiatric disorders in adults in the United States. In: Dohrenwend BP et al., *Mental illness in the United States: epidemiologic estimates*. New York, Praeger.

Link BG et al. (1986) Socio-economic status and schizophrenia: noisome occupational characteristics as a risk factor. *American sociological review*, 51: 242–258.

Lipkowitz MH, Idupuganti S (1985) Diagnosing schizophrenia in 1982: the effect of DSM-III. *American journal of psychiatry*, 142: 634–637.

Loranger AW (1990) The impact of DSM-III on diagnostic practice in a University Hospital. *Archives of general psychiatry*, 47: 672–675.

Mabry CC (1990) Phenylketonuria: contemporary screening and diagnosis. *Annals of clinical and laboratory science*, 20: 392–397.

Malzberg B (1969) Are immigrants psychologically disturbed? In: Plog SC, Edgerton RB, eds. *Changing perspectives in mental illness*, New York, Holt, Rinehart & Winston, pp. 395–421.

Manderscheid RW, Sonnenschein MA, eds. (1990) *Mental health, United States, 1990*. Washington, Government Printing Office (DHHS Pub. No. (ADM) 90–1708).

Marder SR et al. (1979) Predicting drug-free improvement in schizophrenic psychosis. *Archives of general psychiatry*, 36: 1080–1085.

Masterson E, O'Shea B (1984) Smoking and malignancy in schizophrenia. *British journal of psychiatry*, 145: 429–432.

Mavreas VG, Bebbington P (1987) Psychiatric morbidity in London's Greek-Cypriot immigrant community. *Social psychiatry*, 22: 150–159.

Mayer-Gross W (1948) Mental health survey in a rural area. *Eugenics review*, 40: 140–148.

McGlashan TH, Fenton WS (1991) Classical subtypes for schizophrenia. *Schizophrenia bulletin*, 17: 609–623.

McGorry PD et al. (1990) The Royal Park Hospital Multidiagnostic Instrument for

Psychosis: a comprehensive assessment procedure for the acute psychotic episode. I. Rationale and review. *Schizophrenia bulletin*, 16: 501–515.

McGovern D, Cope RV (1987) First psychiatric admission rate of first and second generation Afro-Caribbeans. *Social psychiatry*, 22: 139–149.

McNeil TF (1987) Perinatal influences in the development of schizophrenia. In: Helmchen H, Henn FA, *Biological perspectives of schizophrenia*, New York, John Wiley, pp. 125–138.

McNeil T et al. (1975) Birth rates of schizophrenics following relatively warm versus relatively cool summers. *Archiv für Psychiatrie und Nervenkrankheiten*, 221: 1–10.

McNeil TF et al. (1993) Head circumference in "preschizophrenic" and control neonates. *British journal of psychiatry*, 162: 517–523.

Mednick SA et al. (1987) The Copenhagen high-risk project, 1962-86. *Schizophrenia bulletin*, 13: 485–495.

Mednick SA et al. (1988) Adult schizophrenia following prenatal exposure to an influenza epidemic. *Archives of general psychiatry*, 45: 189–192.

Mellor CS (1982) The present status of first-rank symptoms. *British journal of psychiatry*, 140: 423–424.

Mellsop GW et al. (1991) Reliability of the draft diagnostic criteria for research of ICD-10 in comparison with ICD-10 and DSM-III-R. *Acta psychiatrica scandinavica*, 84: 332–335.

Mortensen PB et al. (1991) Is schizophrenia disappearing? *European archives of psychiatry and clinical neurosciences*, 240: 374.

Mukasa H et al. (1941) Ergebnisse der Geisteskrankenzahlung in einen japanischen Inzuchtgebieten. I. Mitteilung. *Japanese journal of health and human ecology*, 9: 355–397.

Müller HG, Kleider W (1990) A hypothesis on the abnormal seasonality of schizophrenic births. *European archives of psychiatry and neurological sciences*, 239: 331–334.

Munk-Jørgensen P (1986) Decreasing first-admission rates of schizophrenia among males in Denmark from 1970 to 1984. *Acta psychiatrica scandinavica*, 73: 645–650.

Munk-Jørgensen P (1987a) Decreasing rates of diagnoses of schizophrenia in Denmark. *Acta psychiatrica scandinavica*, 76: 333–336 (letter).

Munk-Jørgensen P (1987b) Why has the incidence of schizophrenia in Danish psychiatric institutions decreased since 1970? *Acta psychiatrica scandinavica*, 75: 62–68.

Munk-Jørgensen P, Jørgensen P (1986) Decreasing rates of first-admission diagnoses of schizophrenia among females in Denmark from 1970 to 1984. *Acta psychiatrica scandinavica*, 74: 379–383.

Munk-Jørgensen P, Mortensen PB (1992). Incidence and other aspects of the epidemiology of schizophrenia in Denmark, 1971–1987. *British journal of psychiatry*, 161: 489–495.

Murphy HBM, Lemieux M (1967) Quelques considérations sur le taux élevé de schizophrénie dans un type de communauté canadienne-française. *Canadian Psychiatric Association journal*, 12: S71–S81.

Murphy HBM, Taumoepeau BM (1980) Traditionalism and mental health in the South Pacific: a re-examination of an old hypothesis. *Psychological medicine*, 10: 471–482.

Murray RM et al. (1991) Reply: The incidence of schizophrenia and of causal environmental factors varies in time and place. *European archives of psychiatry and clinical neuroscience*, 240: 377–378.

Murthy RS et al. (1978) Mentally ill in a rural community: some initial experiences in case identification and management. *Indian journal of psychiatry*, 20: 143–147.

Myers JK et al. (1984) Six month prevalences of psychiatric disorders in three sites. *Archives of general psychiatry*, 41: 959–967.

Nandi DN et al. (1975) Psychiatric disorders in a rural community in West Bengal: an epidemiological study. *Indian journal of psychiatry*, 17: 87–99.

Nandi DN et al. (1980) Socio-economic status and mental morbidity in central tribes and castes in India: a cross-cultural study. *British journal of psychiatry*, 136: 73–85.

Nazareth I et al. (1993) Care of schizophrenia in general practice. *British medical journal*, 307: 910.

Nielsen J (1976) The Samsö project from 1957 to 1974. *Acta psychiatrica scandinavica*, 54: 198–222.

Nielsen J, Nielsen JA (1977) A census study of mental illness in Samsö. *Psychological medicine*, 7: 491–503.

Ní Nualláin M et al. (1987) Incidence of schizophrenia in Ireland. *Psychological medicine*, 17: 943–948.

Norman MG, Malla AK (1993) Stressful life events and schizophrenia. I: A review of the research. *British journal of psychiatry*, 162: 161–166.

Norris V (1959) *Mental illness in London*. London, Chapman & Hall (Maudsley Monograph no. 6).

North AF, MacDonald HM (1977) Why are neonatal mortality rates lower in small black infants of similar birth weights? *Journal of pediatrics*, 90: 809–810.

O'Callaghan E et al. (1991) Season of birth in schizophrenia: evidence for confinement of an excess of winter births to patients without a family history of mental disorder. *British journal of psychiatry*, 158: 764–769.

O'Callaghan E et al. (1991) Schizophrenia after prenatal exposure to 1957 A2 influenza epidemic. *Lancet*, 337: 1248–1250.

O'Connor A, Walsh D (1991) *Activities of Irish psychiatric hospitals and units 1988*. Dublin, The Health Research Board.

Ödegaard Ö (1932) Immigration and insanity: a study of mental disease among the Norwegian-born population in Minnesota. *Acta psychiatrica scandinavica*, Suppl. 4.

Ödegaard Ö (1946) A statistical investigation of the incidence of mental disorder in Norway. *Psychiatric quarterly*, 20: 381–401.

Ödegaard Ö (1956) The incidence of psychoses in various occupations. *International journal of social psychiatry*, 2: 85–104.

Ödegaard Ö (1960) A statistical study of factors influencing discharge from psychiatric hospitals. *Journal of mental science*, 106: 1124–1133.

Ödegaard Ö (1971) Hospitalized psychoses in Norway: time trends 1926–1965. *Social psychiatry*, 6: 53–58.

Ödegaard Ö (1974) Season of birth in the general population and in patients with mental disorder in Norway. *British journal of psychiatry*, 125: 397–405.

Odejide AO et al. (1989) Psychiatry in Africa: an overview. *American journal of psychiatry*, 146: 708–716.

O'Hare A et al. (1980) Seasonality of schizophrenic births in Ireland. *British journal of psychiatry*, 137: 74–77.

Ogino R, Nagao S (1943) Über die ortlichen Verschiedenheiten der erbpsychiatrischen Bevölkerungsbelastungen. I. Die erblichen Besonderheiten einer Inzuchtinsel in den Iejima-Inselgruppen. *Psychiatria et neurologia japonica*, 47: 529–536.

Okabe S (1957) Psychiatric and demographic census in the districts of consanguinity. *Psychiatria et neurologia japonica*, 59: 663–676.

Ouspenskaya LY (1978) Problems of methodology of comparative epidemiological studies and the characteristics of prevalence of schizophrenia in various areas of the country. *Zhurnal nevropatologii psikjatrii*, 78: 724–748.

Parker G, Balza B (1977) Season of birth and schizophrenia – an equatorial study. *Acta psychiatrica scandinavica*, 56: 143–146.

Parker G, Neilson M (1976) Mental disorder and season of birth – a southern hemisphere study. *British journal of psychiatry*, 129: 355–361.

Parker G et al. (1985) Changes in the diagnoses of the functional psychoses associated with the introduction of lithium. *British journal of psychiatry*, 146: 377–382.

Parkes CM et al. (1962) The general practitioner and the schizophrenic patient. *British medical journal*, ii: 972–976.

Parnas J et al. (1982) Perinatal complications and clinical outcome within the schizophrenia spectrum. *British journal of psychiatry*, 140: 416–420.

Pasamanick B (1986) Seasonality of schizophrenic births. *American journal of orthopsychiatry*, 56: 168–169.

Phillips L (1953) Case history data and prognosis in schizophrenia. *Journal of nervous and mental disease*, 117: 515–525.

Pichot P (1990) The diagnosis and classification of mental disorders in the French-speaking countries: background, current values and comparison with other classifications. In: Sartorius N et al., eds. *Sources and traditions of classification in psychiatry*. Bern, Hogrefe & Huber, pp. 7–57.

Pollack ES et al. (1964) Socio-economic and family characteristics of patients admitted to psychiatric services. *American journal of public health*, 54: 506–518.

Pope HG, Lipinski JF (1978) Diagnosis in schizophrenia and manic-depressive illness: a reassessment of the specificity of 'schizophrenic' symptoms in the light of current research. *Archives of general psychiatry*, 35: 811–828.

Preiser M, Jeffrey W (1979) Schizophrenic patients and Schneiderian first-rank symptoms. *American journal of psychiatry*, 136: 323–326.

Primrose EJR (1962) *Psychological illness: a community study*. London, Tavistock.

Prince MJ, Phelan MC (1990) Trends in schizophrenia. *Lancet*, 335: 851–852 (letter).

Pull CB, Wittchen HU (1991) CIDI, SCAN and IPDE: structured diagnostic interviews for ICD-10 and DSM-III-R. *European psychiatry*, 6: 277–285.

Pulver AE et al. (1983) Risk factors in schizophrenia: season of birth in Maryland, U.S.A. *British journal of psychiatry*, 143: 389–396.

Pulver AE et al. (1992) Risk factors for schizophrenia. Season of birth, gender and familial risk. *British journal of psychiatry*, 160: 65–71.

Rajkumar S et al. (1991) Schizophrenia Research Foundation (India), Madras, India. Cited in: Eaton WW (1991) Update on the epidemiology of schizophrenia. *Epidemiologic reviews*, 13: 320–328.

Regier DA et al. (1990) Comorbidity of mental disorders with alcohol and other drug abuse. *Journal of the American Medical Association*, 264: 2511–2518.

Reveley AM et al. (1982) Cerebral ventricular size in twins discordant for schizophrenia. *Lancet*, i: 540–541.

Riecher-Rössler A et al. (1992) Is age of onset in schizophrenia influenced by marital status? *Social psychiatry and psychiatric epidemiology*, 27: 122–128.

Rin H, Lin T (1962) Mental illness among Formosan aborigines as compared with the Chinese in Taiwan. *Journal of mental science*, 108: 134–146.

Robins LN et al. (1981) National Institute of Mental Health Diagnostic Interview Schedule: its history, characteristics, and validity. *Archives of general psychiatry*, 39: 381–389.

Robins LN et al. (1988) The Composite International Diagnostic Interview. *Archives of general psychiatry*, 45: 1069–1076.

Roger WF (1950) A comparative study of the Wakefield prison population in 1948. I. *British journal of delinquency*, 1: 15–28.

Roth LH, Ervin FR (1971) Psychiatric care of federal prisoners. *American journal of psychiatry*, 128: 424–430.

Roth WF, Luton FH (1943) The mental health program in Tennessee. *American journal of psychiatry*, 99: 662–675.

Rotstein VT (1977) Material from a psychiatric survey of sample groups from the adult population in several areas of the USSR. *Zhurnal nevropatologii psikijatrii*, 77: 569–574.

Roy C et al. (1970) The prevalence of mental disorders among Saskatchewan Indians. *Journal of cross-cultural psychology*, 1: 383–392.

Sacchetti E et al. (1992) The brain damage hypothesis of the seasonality of births in schizophrenia and major affective disorders: evidence from computerized tomography. *British journal of psychiatry*, 160: 390–397.

Sartorius N et al. (1987) Course of schizophrenia in different countries: some results of a WHO International Comparative 5-year Follow-up Study. In: Häfner H, Gattaz WF, Janzarik W, eds. *Search for the causes of schizophrenia*. Berlin, Springer-Verlag, pp. 107–113.

Sartorius N et al. (1993) Progress towards achieving a common language in psychiatry: results from the ICD-10 clinical field trial of the clinical guidelines accompanying the WHO classification of mental and behavioural disorders in the ICD-10. *Archives of general psychiatry*, 50: 115–124.

Sass H (1987) The classification of schizophrenia in the different diagnostic systems. In: Häfner H, Gattaz WF, Janzarik W, eds. *Search for the causes of schizophrenia*. Berlin, Springer-Verlag, pp. 19–43.

Sato I (1966) Seishin-byōin no tachiba kara. *Seishin igaku*, 8: 6–10.

Schroeder CW (1942) Mental disorders in cities. *American journal of sociology*, 48: 40–48.

Schneider K (1959) *Clinical psychopathology*. New York, Grune & Stratton.

Schulberg HC et al. (1985) Assessing depression in primary medical and psychiatric practices. *Archives of general psychiatry*, 42: 1164–1170.

Scull A (1979) *Museums of madness: the social organization of insanity in nineteenth-century England*. London, Allen Lane.

Seeman M (1982) Gender differences in schizophrenia. *Canadian journal of psychiatry*, 27: 107–112.

Selten JPCJ, Slaets JPJ (1994) Evidence against maternal influenza as a risk factor for schizophrenia. *British journal of psychiatry*, 164: 674–676.

Sethi BB et al. (1967) 300 urban families: a psychiatric study. *Indian journal of psychiatry*, 9: 280–302.

Sethi BB et al. (1972a) Migration and mental health. *Indian journal of psychiatry*, 14: 115–121.

Sethi BB et al. (1972b) A psychiatric survey of 500 rural families. *Indian journal of psychiatry*, 14: 183–196.

Sethi BB et al. (1974) Mental health and urban life: a study of 850 families. *British journal of psychiatry*, 124: 243–246.

Sham PC et al. (1992) Schizophrenia following pre-natal exposure to influenza epidemics between 1939 and 1960. *British journal of psychiatry*, 160: 461–466.

Sham PC et al. (1993) Risk of schizophrenia and age difference with older siblings. Evidence for a maternal viral infection hypothesis? *British journal of psychiatry*, 163: 627–633.

Shen Yucun et al. (1981) Investigations of mental disorders in Beijing suburban district. *Chinese medical journal*, 94: 153–156.

Shen Yucun et al. (1988) A survey of mental disorders in a suburb of Beijing. *International journal of mental health*, 16: 75–80.

Shepherd M (1957) *A study of the major psychoses in an English county.* London, Chapman & Hall (Maudsley Monograph No. 3).

Shepherd M et al. (1966) *Psychiatric illness in general practice.* London, Oxford University Press.

Shepherd M et al. (1989) The natural history of schizophrenia: a five-year follow-up study of outcome and prediction in a representative sample of schizophrenics. *Psychological medicine*, 15 (Suppl.): 1–46

Shibata Y et al. (1975) A psychiatric study on mental disorders in an isolated island. *Clinical psychiatry*, 17: 907–921.

Shibata Y et al. (1978) A psychiatric and socio-medical study on schizophrenics in an isolated island in Yamaguchi Prefecture. *Clinical psychiatry*, 20: 843–852.

Shimura M et al. (1977) Season of birth of schizophrenia in Tokyo, Japan. *Acta psychiatrica scandinavica*, 55: 225–232.

Sikanerty T, Eaton WW (1984) Prevalence of schizophrenia in the Labadi district of Ghana. *Acta psychiatrica scandinavica*, 69: 156–161.

Silverstein ML, Harrow M (1978) First-rank symptoms in the post-acute schizophrenic: a followup study. *American journal of psychiatry*, 135: 1481–1486.

Sjögren T (1948) Genetic-statistical and psychiatric investigations of a West Swedish population. *Acta psychiatrica et neurologica scandinavica*, 52 (Suppl.).

Spitzer RL et al. (1977) *Research diagnostic criteria*. 3rd ed. New York, New York State Psychiatric Institute.

Spitzer RL, Endicott J (1978) *NIMH Clinical Research Branch Collaborative Program on the Psychology of Depression: schedule for affective disorders and schizophrenia*. 3rd ed. New York, New York State Psychiatric Institute, Biometrics Research Division.

Spitzer RL, Fleiss JL (1974) A reanalysis of the reliability of psychiatric diagnosis. *British journal of psychology*, 125: 341–347.

Spitzer RL, Williams JBW (1985) *Structured clinical interview for DSM-III*. New York, New York State Psychiatric Institute, Biometrics Research Division.

Stabenau JR, Pollin W (1967) Early characteristics of MZ twins discordant for schizophrenia. *Archives of general psychiatry*, 17: 723–734.

Stefánsson JG et al. (1991) Lifetime prevalence of specific mental disorders among people born in Iceland in 1931. *Acta psychiatrica scandinavica*, 84: 142–149.

Stein L (1957) "Social class" gradient in schizophrenia. *British journal of preventive and social medicine*, 11: 181–195.

Stephens JH et al. (1966) Prognostic factors in recovered and deteriorated schizophrenics. *American journal of psychiatry*, 122: 1116–1121.

Stevens J (1987) Brief psychoses: do they contribute to the good prognosis and equal prevalence of schizophrenia in developing countries? *British journal of psychiatry*, 151: 393–396.

Stevens JR (1982) Neuropathology of schizophrenia. *Archives of general psychiatry*, 39: 1131–1139.

Stoll AL et al. (1993) Shifts in diagnostic frequencies of schizophrenia and major affective disorders at six North American psychiatric hospitals, 1972–1988. *American journal of psychiatry*, 150: 1668–1673.

Strauss JS, Gift TE (1977) Choosing an approach for diagnosing schizophrenia. *Archives of general psychiatry*, 34: 1248–1253.

Strömgren E (1938) Beiträge zur psychiatrischen Erblehre. *Acta psychiatrica et neurologica scandinavica*, (Suppl. 19).

Strömgren E (1987) Changes in the incidence of schizophrenia. *British journal of psychiatry*, 150: 1–7.

Strömgren E et al. (1989) Discussion. *Acta psychiatrica scandinavica* (Suppl. 348): 167–178.

Suddath RL et al. (1989) Quantitative magnetic resonance imaging in twin pairs discordant for schizophrenia. *Schizophrenia research*, 2: 129.

Sundby P, Nyhus P (1963) Major and minor psychiatric disorders in males in Oslo: an epidemiological study. *Acta psychiatrica scandinavica*, 39: 519–547.

Surya NC et al. (1964) Mental morbidity in Pondicherry (1962–1963). *Transaction (All Indian Insitute of Mental Health, Bangalore)*, 4: 50–61.

Takei N et al. (1994) Prenatal exposure to influenza and the development of schizophrenia: is the effect confined to females? *American journal of psychiatry*, 151: 117–119.

Taylor MA (1972) Schneiderian first-rank symptoms and clinical prognostic features in schizophrenia. *Archives of general psychiatry*, 26: 64–67.

Taylor MA, Abrams R (1975) The phenomenology of mania: a new look at some old patients. *Archives of general psychiatry*, 29: 520–522.

Temkov I et al. (1980) Use of reported prevalence data in cross-national comparisons of psychiatric morbidity. *Social psychiatry*, 3: 111–117.

ten Horn GHMM et al., eds. (1986) *Psychiatric case registers in public health*. Amsterdam, Elsevier.

Teplin LA (1990) The prevalence of severe mental disorder among male urban jail detainees: comparison with the Epidemiologic Catchment Area Program. *American journal of public health*, 80: 663–669.

Terry PB et al. (1987) Ethnic differences in incidence of very low birthweight and neonatal deaths among normally formed infants. *Archives of disease in childhood*, 62: 709–711.

Thacore VR et al. (1975) Psychiatric morbidity in a north Indian community. *British journal of psychiatry*, 126: 364–369.

Thomas CS et al. (1993) Psychiatric morbidity and compulsory admissions amongst whites, Afro-Caribbeans, and Asians in central Manchester. *British journal of psychiatry*, 163: 91–99.

Thurnam J (1845) *Observations and essays on the statistics of insanity*. London, Simpkins, Marshall.

Tien AY (1991) Distribution of hallucinations in the population. *Social psychiatry*, 26: 287–292.

Tien AY, Eaton WW (1992) Psychopathologic precursors and sociodemographic risk factors for the schizophrenia syndrome. *Archives of general psychiatry*, 49: 37–46.

Tienari P et al. (1987) Genetic and psychosocial factors in schizophrenia: the Finnish adoptive family study. *Schizophrenia bulletin*, 13: 477–484.

Torrey EF (1980) *Schizophrenia and civilization*. New York, Jason Aronson.

Torrey EF (1987) Prevalence studies in schizophrenia. *British journal of psychiatry*, 150: 598–608.

Torrey EF (1989) Schizophrenia: fixed incidence or fixed thinking? *Psychological medicine*, 19: 285–287.

Torrey EF et al. (1977) Seasonality of schizophrenic births in the United States. *Archives of general psychiatry*, 34: 1065–1070.

Torrey EF et al. (1984) Endemic psychosis in western Ireland. *American journal of psychiatry*, 141: 966–969.

Torrey EF et al. (1988) Schizophrenic births and viral diseases in two states. *Schizophrenia research*, 1: 73–77.

Tramer M (1929) Über die biologische Bedeutung des Geburtsmonates, insbesondere für die Psychoseerkrankung. *Schweizer Archiv für Neurologie und Psychiatrie*, 24: 17–24.

Tsugawa B (1942) Daitoshi ni okeru seishin-shikkan no hassei-hindo ni kansuru kenkyū. *Seishin shinnkei gaku zasshi*, 47: 204.

Turner RJ, Wagenfeld MO (1967) Occupational mobility and schizophrenia: an assessment of the social causation and social selection hypotheses. *American sociological review*, 32: 104–113.

Uchimura Y (1940) Hachijō-jima ni okeru seishin-shikkan no hassei-hindo ni kansuru kenkyū. *Minzoku eisei*, 10: 1.

Uchimura Y et al. (1942) Eine weitere vergleichend psychiatrische und erbpathologische Untersuchung auf einer japanischen Insel. *Japanese journal of health and human ecology*, 10: 1–151.

Väisänen E (1975) Psychiatric disorders in Finland. *Acta psychiatrica scandinavica* (Suppl. 263): 22–33.

Van Horn JD, McManus IC (1992) Ventricular enlargement in schizophrenia: a meta-analysis of studies of the ventricle: brain ratio (VBR). *British journal of psychiatry*, 160: 687–697.

van Os J et al. (1993) Schizophrenia sans frontières: concepts of schizophrenia among French and British psychiatrists. *British medical journal*, 307: 489–492.

Varga E (1966) *Changes in the symptomatology of psychotic patterns*. Budapest, Akademiai Kiado.

Vazquez-Barquero JL et al. (1987) A community mental health survey in Cantabria: a general description of morbidity. *Psychological medicine*, 17: 227–241.

Verghese A et al. (1973) A social and psychiatric study of a representative group of families in Vellore town. *Indian journal of medical research*, 61: 608–620.

Videbech T et al. (1974) Endogenous psychoses and season of birth. *Acta psychiatrica scandinavica*, 50: 202–218.

Von Korff M et al. (1991) Prevalence of treated and untreated DSM-III schizophrenia. Results of a two-stage community survey. *Journal of nervous and mental disease*, 173: 577–581.

Waddington JL, Youssef HA (1994) Evidence for a gender-specific decline in the rate of schizophrenia in rural Ireland over a 50-year period. *British journal of psychiatry*, 164: 171–176.

Walker EF, Lewine RRJ (1993) Sampling biases in studies of gender and schizophrenia. *Schizophrenia bulletin*, 19: 1–7.

Walsh D (1969) Mental illness in Dublin: first admissions. *British journal of psychiatry*, 115: 449–456.

Walsh D (1976) Two and two make five: multifactoriogenesis in mental illness in Ireland. *Journal of the Irish Medical Association*, 69: 417–422.

Walsh D, Walsh B (1970) Mental illness in the Republic of Ireland: first admissions. *Journal of the Irish Medical Association*, 63: 365–370.

Walsh D et al. (1980) The treated prevalence of mental illness in the Republic of Ireland: the three county case register study. *Psychological medicine*, 10: 465–470.

Warner R (1983) Recovery from schizophrenia in the Third World. *Psychiatry*, 46: 197–212.

Warner R (1985) *Recovery from schizophrenia: psychiatry and political economy*. London, Routledge & Kegan Paul.

Warner R (1994) *Recovery from schizophrenia*, 2nd ed. London, Routledge.

Warthen FJ et al. (1967) Diagnosed schizophrenia in Maryland. In: Monroe RR et al., eds. *Psychiatric epidemiology and mental health planning*, Washington, American Psychiatric Press, pp. 149–170.

Watson CG et al. (1984) Schizophrenic birth seasonality in relation to the incidence of infectious diseases and temperature extremes. *Archives of general psychiatry*, 41: 85–90.

Weinberger DR, Kleinman JE (1986) Observations on the brain in schizophrenia. In: Frances AJ, Hales RE, eds. *Psychiatry update: American Psychiatric Association annual review. Volume 5*. Washington, DC, American Psychiatric Press, pp. 42–67.

Weissman MM, Myers JK (1980) Psychiatric disorders in a U.S. community. The application of research diagnostic criteria to a resurveyed community sample. *Acta psychiatrica scandinavica*, 62: 99–111.

Wells EJ et al. (1989) Christchurch psychiatric epidemiology study. Part I: Methodology and lifetime prevalence for specific psychiatric disorders. *Australian and New Zealand journal of psychiatry*, 23: 315–326.

Wender PH et al. (1974) Cross-fostering: a research strategy for clarifying the role of genetic and experiential factors in the etiology of schizophrenia. *Archives of general psychiatry*, 30: 121–128.

Wessely S et al. (1991) Schizophrenia and Afro-Caribbeans: a case-control study. *British journal of psychiatry*, 159: 795–801.

WHO (1973) *The International Pilot Study of Schizophrenia*. Geneva, World Health Organization (WHO Offset Publication, No. 2).

WHO (1979) *Schizophrenia: an international follow-up study*. Chichester, Wiley.

WHO (1992) *The ICD-10 Classification of Mental and Behavioural Disorders. Clinical descriptions and diagnostic guidelines*. Geneva, World Health Organization.

Widerlov B et al. (1989) Epidemiology of long-term functional psychosis in three different areas in Stockholm County. *Acta psychiatrica scandinavica*, 80: 40–46.

Wig NN, Parhee R (1989) Acute and transient psychoses: a view from the developing countries. In: Mezzich JE, von Cranach M, eds. *International classification in psychiatry: unity and diversity*, Cambridge, Cambridge University Press, pp. 115–121.

Wijesinghe CP et al. (1978) Survey of psychiatric morbidity in a semi-urban population in Sri Lanka. *Acta psychiatrica scandinavica*, 58: 413–441.

Wing JK, Fryers T (1976) *Statistics from the Camberwell and Salford psychiatric registers 1964–1974*. London, Institute of Psychiatry.

Wing JK et al. (1967) The use of psychiatric services in three urban areas: an international case register study. *Social psychiatry*, 2: 158–167.

Wing JK et al. (1974) *Measurement and diagnosis of psychiatric symptoms*. London, Cambridge University Press.

Wing JK et al. (1990) SCAN: Schedules for clinical assessment in neuropsychiatry. *Archives of general psychiatry*, 47: 589–593.

Wittchen HU et al. (1991) Cross-cultural feasibility, reliability and sources of variance of the Composite International Diagnostic Interview (CIDI). *British journal of psychiatry*, 159: 645–653.

Wulff E (1967) Psychiatrischer Bericht aus Vietnam. In: Petrilowitsch N, ed. *Beitrage zur vergleichenden Psychiatrie*. Basel, Karger, pp. 1–84.

Youssef HA et al. (1991) Evidence for geographical variations in the prevalence of schizophrenia in rural Ireland. *Archives of general psychiatry*, 48: 254–258.

Zharikov NM (1968) Epidemiological study of mental illness in the U.S.S.R. *Social psychiatry*, 3: 135–138.

Zimmerman-Tansella C et al. (1985) Bringing into action the psychiatric reform in South-Verona: a five year experience. *Acta psychiatrica scandinavica*, 316 (Suppl.): 71–86.

Clinical descriptions and diagnostic guidelines[1]

F20–F29 Schizophrenia, schizotypal and delusional disorders

Schizophrenia is the commonest and most important disorder of this group. Schizotypal disorder possesses many of the characteristic features of schizophrenic disorders and is probably genetically related to them; however, the hallucinations, delusions, and gross behavioural disturbances of schizophrenia itself are absent and so this disorder does not always come to medical attention. Most of the delusional disorders are probably unrelated to schizophrenia, although they may be difficult to distinguish clinically, particularly in their early stages. They form a heterogeneous and poorly understood collection of disorders, which can conveniently be divided according to their typical duration into a group of persistent delusional disorders and a larger group of acute and transient psychotic disorders. The latter appear to be particularly common in developing countries. The subdivisions listed here should be regarded as provisional. Schizoaffective disorders have been retained in this section in spite of their controversial nature.

F20 Schizophrenia

The schizophrenic disorders are characterized in general by fundamental and characteristic distortions of thinking and perception, and by inappropriate or blunted affect. Clear consciousness and intellectual capacity are usually maintained, although certain cognitive deficits may evolve in the course of time. The disturbance involves the most basic functions that give the normal person a feeling of individuality, uniqueness, and self-direction. The most intimate thoughts, feelings, and acts are often felt to be known to or shared by others, and explanatory delusions may develop, to the effect that natural or supernatural forces are at work to influence the afflicted individual's thoughts and actions in ways that are often bizarre. The individual may see himself or herself as the pivot of all that happens. Hallucinations, especially auditory, are common and may comment on the individual's behaviour or thoughts. Perception is frequently disturbed in other ways: colours or sounds may seem unduly vivid or altered in quality, and irrelevant features of ordinary things

---

[1] Reproduced from: *The ICD-10 Classification of Mental and Behavioural Disorders: clinical descriptions and diagnostic guidelines.* Geneva, World Health Organization, 1992, pp. 86–109.

may appear more important than the whole object or situation. Perplexity is also common early on and frequently leads to a belief that everyday situations possess a special, usually sinister, meaning intended uniquely for the individual. In the characteristic schizophrenic disturbance of thinking, peripheral and irrelevant features of a total concept, which are inhibited in normal directed mental activity, are brought to the fore and utilized in place of those that are relevant and appropriate to the situation. Thus thinking becomes vague, elliptical, and obscure, and its expression in speech sometimes incomprehensible. Breaks and interpolations in the train of thought are frequent, and thoughts may seem to be withdrawn by some outside agency. Mood is characteristically shallow, capricious, or incongruous. Ambivalence and disturbance of volition may appear as inertia, negativism, or stupor. Catatonia may be present. The onset may be acute, with seriously disturbed behaviour, or insidious, with a gradual development of odd ideas and conduct. The course of the disorder shows equally great variation and is by no means inevitably chronic or deteriorating (the course is specified by five-character categories). In a proportion of cases, which may vary in different cultures and populations, the outcome is complete, or nearly complete, recovery. The sexes are approximately equally affected but the onset tends to be later in women.

Although no strictly pathognomonic symptoms can be identified, for practical purposes it is useful to divide the above symptoms into groups that have special importance for the diagnosis and often occur together, such as:

(a) thought echo, thought insertion or withdrawal, and thought broadcasting;

(b) delusions of control, influence, or passivity, clearly referred to body or limb movements or specific thoughts, actions, or sensations; delusional perception;

(c) hallucinatory voices giving a running commentary on the patient's behaviour, or discussing the patient among themselves, or other types of hallucinatory voices coming from some part of the body;

(d) persistent delusions of other kinds that are culturally inappropriate and completely impossible, such as religious or political identity, or superhuman powers and abilities (e.g. being able to control the weather, or being in communication with aliens from another world);

(e) persistent hallucinations in any modality, when accompanied either by fleeting or half-formed delusions without clear affective content, or by persistent over-valued ideas, or when occurring every day for weeks or months on end;

(f) breaks or interpolations in the train of thought, resulting in incoherence or irrelevant speech, or neologisms;

(g) catatonic behaviour, such as excitement, posturing, or waxy flexibility, negativism, mutism, and stupor;

(h) "negative" symptoms such as marked apathy, paucity of speech, and blunting or incongruity of emotional responses, usually resulting in social withdrawal and lowering of social performance; it must be clear that these are not due to depression or to neuroleptic medication;

(i) a significant and consistent change in the overall quality of some aspects of personal behaviour, manifest as loss of interest, aimlessness, idleness, a self-absorbed attitude, and social withdrawal.

Diagnostic guidelines

The normal requirement for a diagnosis of schizophrenia is that a minimum of one very clear symptom (and usually two or more if less clear-cut) belonging to any one of the groups listed as (a) to (d) above, or symptoms from at least two of the groups referred to as (e) to (h), should have been clearly present for most of the time *during a period of 1 month or more.* Conditions meeting such symptomatic requirements but of duration less than 1 month (whether treated or not) should be diagnosed in the first instance as acute schizophrenia-like psychotic disorder (F23.2) and reclassified as schizophrenia if the symptoms persist for longer periods.

Viewed retrospectively, it may be clear that a prodromal phase in which symptoms and behaviour, such as loss of interest in work, social activities, and personal appearance and hygiene, together with generalized anxiety and mild degrees of depression and preoccupation, preceded the onset of psychotic symptoms by weeks or even months. Because of the difficulty in timing onset, the 1-month duration criterion applies only to the specific symptoms listed above and not to any prodromal nonpsychotic phase.

The diagnosis of schizophrenia should not be made in the presence of extensive depressive or manic symptoms unless it is clear that schizophrenic symptoms antedated the affective disturbance. If both schizophrenic and affective symptoms develop together and are evenly balanced, the diagnosis of schizoaffective disorder (F25.–) should be made, even if the schizophrenic symptoms by themselves would have justified the diagnosis of schizophrenia. Schizophrenia should not be diagnosed in the presence of overt brain disease or during states of drug intoxication or withdrawal. Similar disorders developing in the presence of epilepsy or other brain disease should be coded under F06.2 and those induced by drugs under F1x.5.

Pattern of course

The course of schizophrenic disorders can be classified by using the following five-character codes:

F20.x0 Continuous
F20.x1 Episodic with progressive deficit
F20.x2 Episodic with stable deficit
F20.x3 Episodic remittent
F20.x4 Incomplete remission
F20.x5 Complete remission
F20.x8 Other
F20.x9 Period of observation less than one year

F20.0 Paranoid schizophrenia

This is the commonest type of schizophrenia in most parts of the world. The clinical picture is dominated by relatively stable, often paranoid, delusions, usually accompanied by hallucinations, particularly of the auditory variety, and perceptual disturbances. Disturbances of affect, volition, and speech, and catatonic symptoms, are not prominent.

Examples of the most common paranoid symptoms are:

(a) delusions of persecution, reference, exalted birth, special mission, bodily change, or jealousy;
(b) hallucinatory voices that threaten the patient or give commands, or auditory hallucinations without verbal form, such as whistling, humming, or laughing;
(c) hallucinations of smell or taste, or of sexual or other bodily sensations; visual hallucinations may occur but are rarely predominant.

Thought disorder may be obvious in acute states, but if so it does not prevent the typical delusions or hallucinations from being described clearly. Affect is usually less blunted than in other varieties of schizophrenia, but a minor degree of incongruity is common, as are mood disturbances such as irritability, sudden anger, fearfulness, and suspicion. "Negative" symptoms such as blunting of affect and impaired volition are often present but do not dominate the clinical picture.

The course of paranoid schizophrenia may be episodic, with partial or complete remissions, or chronic. In chronic cases, the florid symptoms persist over years and it is difficult to distinguish discrete episodes. The onset tends to be later than in the hebephrenic and catatonic forms.

Diagnostic guidelines

The general criteria for a diagnosis of schizophrenia (see introduction to F20 above) must be satisfied. In addition, hallucinations and/or delusions must be prominent, and disturbances of affect, volition and speech, and catatonic symptoms must be relatively inconspicuous. The hallucinations will usually be of the kind described in (b) and (c) above. Delusions can be of almost any kind but delusions of control, influence, or passivity, and persecutory beliefs of various kinds are the most characteristic.

Includes: paraphrenic schizophrenia

Differential diagnosis. It is important to exclude epileptic and drug-induced psychoses, and to remember that persecutory delusions might carry little diagnostic weight in people from certain countries or cultures.

Excludes: involutional paranoid state (F22.8)
　　　　　paranoia (F22.0)

F20.1 Hebephrenic schizophrenia

A form of schizophrenia in which affective changes are prominent, delusions and hallucinations fleeting and fragmentary, behaviour irresponsible and unpredictable, and mannerisms common. The mood is shallow and inappropriate and often accompanied by giggling or self-satisfied, self-absorbed smiling, or by a lofty manner, grimaces, mannerisms, pranks, hypochondriacal complaints, and reiterated phrases. Thought is disorganized and speech rambling and incoherent. There is a tendency to remain solitary, and behaviour seems empty of purpose and feeling. This form of schizophrenia usually starts between the ages of 15 and 25 years and tends to have a poor prognosis because of the rapid development of "negative" symptoms, particularly flattening of affect and loss of volition.

In addition, disturbances of affect and volition, and thought disorder are usually prominent. Hallucinations and delusions may be present but are not usually prominent. Drive and determination are lost and goals abandoned, so that the patient's behaviour becomes characteristically aimless and empty of purpose. A superficial and manneristic preoccupation with religion, philosophy, and other abstract themes may add to the listener's difficulty in following the train of thought.

Diagnostic guidelines

The general criteria for a diagnosis of schizophrenia (see introduction to F20 above) must be satisfied. Hebephrenia should normally be diagnosed for the first time only in adolescents or young adults. The premorbid personality is characteristically, but not necessarily, rather shy and solitary. For a confident diagnosis of hebephrenia, a period of 2 or 3 months of continuous observation is usually necessary, in order to ensure that the characteristic behaviours described above are sustained.

Includes: disorganized schizophrenia
        hebephrenia

F20.2 Catatonic schizophrenia

Prominent psychomotor disturbances are essential and dominant features and may alternate between extremes such as hyperkinesis and stupor, or automatic obedience and negativism. Constrained attitudes and postures may be maintained for long periods. Episodes of violent excitement may be a striking feature of the condition.

For reasons that are poorly understood, catatonic schizophrenia is now rarely seen in industrial countries, though it remains common elsewhere. These catatonic phenomena may be combined with a dream-like (oneiroid) state with vivid scenic hallucinations.

Diagnostic guidelines

The general criteria for a diagnosis of schizophrenia (see introduction to F20 above) must be satisfied. Transitory and isolated catatonic symptoms may occur in the context of any other subtype of schizophrenia, but for a diagnosis of catatonic schizophrenia one or more of the following behaviours should dominate the clinical picture:

(a) stupor (marked decrease in reactivity to the environment and in spontaneous movements and activity) or mutism;

(b) excitement (apparently purposeless motor activity, not influenced by external stimuli);

(c) posturing (voluntary assumption and maintenance of inappropriate or bizarre postures);

(d) negativism (an apparently motiveless resistance to all instructions or attempts to be moved, or movement in the opposite direction);

(e) rigidity (maintenance of a rigid posture against efforts to be moved);

(f) waxy flexibility (maintenance of limbs and body in externally imposed positions); and

(g) other symptoms such as command automatism (automatic compliance with instructions), and perseveration of words and phrases.

In uncommunicative patients with behavioural manifestations of catatonic disorder, the diagnosis of schizophrenia may have to be provisional until adequate evidence of the presence of other symptoms is obtained. It is also vital to appreciate that catatonic symptoms are not diagnostic of schizophrenia. A catatonic symptom or symptoms may also be provoked by brain disease, metabolic disturbances, or alcohol and drugs, and may also occur in mood disorders.

Includes: catatonic stupor
schizophrenic catalepsy
schizophrenic catatonia
schizophrenic flexibilitas cerea

F20.3 Undifferentiated schizophrenia

Conditions meeting the general diagnostic criteria for schizophrenia (see introduction to F20 above) but not conforming to any of the above subtypes (F20.0–F20.2), or exhibiting the features of more than one of them without a clear predominance of a particular set of diagnostic characteristics. This rubric should be used only for psychotic conditions (i.e. residual schizophrenia, F20.5, and post-schizophrenic depression, F20.4, are excluded) and after an attempt has been made to classify the condition into one of the three preceding categories.

Diagnostic guidelines

This category should be reserved for disorders that:

(a) meet the diagnostic criteria for schizophrenia;

(b) do not satisfy the criteria for the paranoid, hebephrenic, or catatonic subtypes;

(c) do not satisfy the criteria for residual schizophrenia or post-schizophrenic depression.

Includes: atypical schizophrenia

F20.4 Post-schizophrenic depression

A depressive episode, which may be prolonged, arising in the aftermath of a schizophrenic illness. Some schizophrenic symptoms must still be present but no longer dominate the clinical picture. These persisting schizophrenic symptoms may be "positive" or "negative", though the latter are more common. It is uncertain, and immaterial to the diagnosis, to what extent the depressive symptoms have merely been uncovered by the resolution of earlier psychotic symptoms (rather than being a new development) or are an intrinsic part of schizophrenia rather than a psychological reaction to it. They are rarely sufficiently severe or extensive to meet criteria for a severe depressive episode (F32.2 and F32.3), and it is often difficult to decide which of the patient's symptoms are due to depression and which to neuroleptic medication or to the impaired volition and affective flattening of schizophrenia itself. This depressive disorder is associated with an increased risk of suicide.

Diagnostic guidelines

The diagnosis should be made only if:
(a) the patient has had a schizophrenic illness meeting the general criteria for schizophrenia (see introduction to F20 above) within the past 12 months;
(b) some schizophrenic symptoms are still present; and
(c) the depressive symptoms are prominent and distressing, fulfilling at least the criteria for a depressive episode (F32.–), and have been present for at least 2 weeks.

If the patient no longer has any schizophrenic symptoms, a depressive episode should be diagnosed (F32.–). If schizophrenic symptoms are still florid and prominent, the diagnosis should remain that of the appropriate schizophrenic subtype (F20.0, F20.1, F20.2, or F20.3).

F20.5 Residual schizophrenia

A chronic stage in the development of a schizophrenic disorder in which there has been a clear progression from an early stage (comprising one or more episodes with psychotic symptoms meeting the general criteria for schizophrenia described above) to a later stage characterized by long-term, though not necessarily irreversible, "negative" symptoms.

Diagnostic guidelines

For a confident diagnosis, the following requirements should be met:

(a) prominent "negative" schizophrenic symptoms, i.e. psychomotor slowing, underactivity, blunting of affect, passivity and lack of initiative, poverty of quantity or content of speech, poor nonverbal communication by facial expression, eye contact, voice modulation, and posture, poor self-care and social performance;
(b) evidence in the past of at least one clear-cut psychotic episode meeting the diagnostic criteria for schizophrenia;
(c) a period of *at least 1 year* during which the intensity and frequency of florid

symptoms such as delusions and hallucinations have been minimal or substantially reduced *and* the "negative" schizophrenic syndrome has been present;

(d) absence of dementia or other organic brain disease or disorder, and of chronic depression or institutionalism sufficient to explain the negative impairments.

If adequate information about the patient's previous history cannot be obtained, and it therefore cannot be established that criteria for schizophrenia have been met at some time in the past, it may be necessary to make a provisional diagnosis of residual schizophrenia.

Includes: chronic undifferentiated schizophrenia
"Restzustand"
schizophrenic residual state

F20.6 Simple schizophrenia

An uncommon disorder in which there is an insidious but progressive development of oddities of conduct, inability to meet the demands of society, and decline in total performance. Delusions and hallucinations are not evident, and the disorder is less obviously psychotic than the hebephrenic, paranoid, and catatonic subtypes of schizophrenia. The characteristic "negative" features of residual schizophrenia (e.g. blunting of affect, loss of volition) develop without being preceded by any overt psychotic symptoms. With increasing social impoverishment, vagrancy may ensue and the individual may then become self-absorbed, idle, and aimless.

Diagnostic guidelines

Simple schizophrenia is a difficult diagnosis to make with any confidence because it depends on establishing the slowly progressive development of the characteristic "negative" symptoms of residual schizophrenia (see F20.5 above) without any history of hallucinations, delusions, or other manifestations of an earlier psychotic episode, and with significant changes in personal behaviour, manifest as a marked loss of interest, idleness, and social withdrawal.

Includes: schizophrenia simplex

F20.8 Other schizophrenia

Includes: cenesthopathic schizophrenia
schizophreniform disorder NOS

Excludes: acute schizophrenia-like disorder (F23.2)
cyclic schizophrenia (F25.2)
latent schizophrenia (F23.2)

F20.9 Schizophrenia, unspecified

F21 Schizotypal disorder

A disorder characterized by eccentric behaviour and anomalies of thinking and affect which resemble those seen in schizophrenia, though no definite and characteristic schizophrenic anomalies have occurred at any stage. There is no dominant or typical disturbance, but any of the following may be present:

(a) inappropriate or constricted affect (the individual appears cold and aloof);
(b) behaviour or appearance that is odd, eccentric, or peculiar;
(c) poor rapport with others and a tendency to social withdrawal;
(d) odd beliefs or magical thinking, influencing behaviour and inconsistent with subcultural norms;
(e) suspiciousness or paranoid ideas;
(f) obsessive ruminations without inner resistance, often with dysmorpho-phobic, sexual or aggressive contents;
(g) unusual perceptual experiences including somatosensory (bodily) or other illusions, depersonalization or derealization;
(h) vague, circumstantial, metaphorical, overelaborate, or stereotyped think-ing, manifested by odd speech or in other ways, without gross incoherence;
(i) occasional transient quasi-psychotic episodes with intense illusions, audi-tory or other hallucinations, and delusion-like ideas, usually occurring without external provocation.

The disorder runs a chronic course with fluctuations of intensity. Occa-sionally it evolves into overt schizophrenia. There is no definite onset and its evolution and course are usually those of a personality disorder. It is more common in individuals related to schizophrenics and is believed to be part of the genetic "spectrum" of schizophrenia.

Diagnostic guidelines
This diagnostic rubric is not recommended for general use because it is not clearly demarcated either from simple schizophrenia or from schizoid or paranoid personality disorders. If the term is used, three or four of the typical features listed above should have been present, continuously or episodically, for *at least 2 years*. The individual must never have met criteria for schizophrenia itself. A history of schizophrenia in a first-degree relative gives additional weight to the diagnosis but is not a prerequisite.

Includes: borderline schizophrenia
latent schizophrenia
latent schizophrenic reaction
prepsychotic schizophrenia
prodromal schizophrenia
pseudoneurotic schizophrenia
pseudopsychopathic schizophrenia
schizotypal personality disorder

Excludes: Asperger's syndrome (F84.5)
schizoid personality disorder (F60.1)

F22 Persistent delusional disorders

This group includes a variety of disorders in which long-standing delusions constitute the only, or the most conspicuous, clinical characteristic and which cannot be classified as organic, schizophrenic, or affective. They are probably heterogeneous, and have uncertain relationships to schizophrenia. The relative importance of genetic factors, personality characteristics, and life circumstances in their genesis is uncertain and probably variable.

F22.0 Delusional disorder

This group of disorders is characterized by the development either of a single delusion or of a set of related delusions which are usually persistent and sometimes lifelong. The delusions are highly variable in content. Often they are persecutory, hypochondriacal, or grandiose, but they may be concerned with litigation or jealousy, or express a conviction that the individual's body is misshapen, or that others think that he or she smells or is homosexual. Other psychopathology is characteristically absent, but depressive symptoms may be present intermittently, and olfactory and tactile hallucinations may develop in some cases. Clear and persistent auditory hallucinations (voices), schizophrenic symptoms such as delusions of control and marked blunting of affect, and definite evidence of brain disease are all incompatible with this diagnosis. However, occasional or transitory auditory hallucinations, particularly in elderly patients, do not rule out this diagnosis, provided that they are not typically schizophrenic and form only a small part of the overall clinical picture. Onset is commonly in middle age but sometimes, particularly in the case of beliefs about having a misshapen body, in early adult life. The content of the delusion, and the timing of its emergence, can often be related to the individual's life situation, e.g. persecutory delusions in members of minorities. Apart from actions and attitudes directly related to the delusion or delusional system, affect, speech, and behaviour are normal.

Diagnostic guidelines

Delusions constitute the most conspicuous or the only clinical characteristic. They must be present for at least 3 months and be clearly personal rather than subcultural. Depressive symptoms or even a full-blown depressive episode (F32.–) may be present intermittently, provided that the delusion persists at times when there is no disturbance of mood. There must be no evidence of brain disease, no or only occasional auditory hallucinations, and no history of schizophrenic symptoms (delusions of control, thought broadcasting, etc.).

Includes: paranoia
paranoid psychosis

paranoid state
paraphrenia (late)
sensitiver Beziehungswahn

Excludes: paranoid personality disorder (F60.0)
psychogenic paranoid psychosis (F23.3)
paranoid reaction (F23.3)
paranoid schizophrenia (F20.0)

F22.8 Other persistent delusional disorders

This is a residual category for persistent delusional disorders that do not meet
the criteria for delusional disorder (F22.0). Disorders in which delusions are
accompanied by persistent hallucinatory voices or by schizophrenic symptoms
that are insufficient to meet criteria for schizophrenia (F20.–) should be coded
here. Delusional disorders that have lasted for less than 3 months should,
however, be coded, at least temporarily, under F23.–.

Includes: delusional dysmorphophobia
involutional paranoid state
paranoia querulans

F22.9 Persistent delusional disorder, unspecified

F23 Acute and transient psychotic disorders

Systematic clinical information that would provide definitive guidance on the
classification of acute psychotic disorders is not yet available, and the limited
data and clinical tradition that must therefore be used instead do not give rise to
concepts that can be clearly defined and separated from each other. In the
absence of a tried and tested multiaxial system, the method used here to avoid
diagnostic confusion is to construct a diagnostic sequence that reflects the order
of priority given to selected key features of the disorder. The order of priority
used here is:

(a) an acute onset (within 2 weeks) as the defining feature of the whole group;
(b) the presence of typical syndromes;
(c) the presence of associated acute stress.

The classification is nevertheless arranged so that those who do not agree
with this order of priority can still identify acute psychotic disorders with each
of these specified features.

It is also recommended that whenever possible a further subdivision of onset
be used, if applicable, for all the disorders of this group. *Acute onset* is defined as a
change from a state without psychotic features to a clearly abnormal psychotic
state, within a period of 2 weeks or less. There is some evidence that acute onset
is associated with a good outcome, and it may be that the more abrupt the
onset, the better the outcome. It is therefore recommended that, whenever
appropriate, *abrupt onset* (within 48 hours or less) be specified.

The *typical syndromes* that have been selected are first, the rapidly changing and variable state, called here "polymorphic", that has been given prominence in acute psychotic states in several countries, and second, the presence of typical schizophrenic symptoms.

Associated acute stress can also be specified, with a fifth character if desired, in view of its traditional linkage with acute psychosis. The limited evidence available, however, indicates that a substantial proportion of acute psychotic disorders arise without associated stress, and provision has therefore been made for the presence or the absence of stress to be recorded. Associated acute stress is taken to mean that the first psychotic symptoms occur within about 2 weeks of one or more events that would be regarded as stressful to most people in similar circumstances, within the culture of the person concerned. Typical events would be bereavement, unexpected loss of partner or job, marriage, or the psychological trauma of combat, terrorism, and torture. Long-standing difficulties or problems should not be included as a source of stress in this context.

Complete recovery usually occurs within 2 to 3 months, often within a few weeks or even days, and only a small proportion of patients with these disorders develop persistent and disabling states. Unfortunately, the present state of knowledge does not allow the early prediction of that small proportion of patients who will not recover rapidly.

These clinical descriptions and diagnostic guidelines are written on the assumption that they will be used by clinicians who may need to make a diagnosis when having to assess and treat patients within a few days or weeks of the onset of the disorder, not knowing how long the disorder will last. A number of reminders about the time limits and transition from one disorder to another have therefore been included, so as to alert those recording the diagnosis to the need to keep them up to date.

The nomenclature of these acute disorders is as uncertain as their nosological status, but an attempt has been made to use simple and familiar terms. "Psychotic disorder" is used as a term of convenience for all the members of this group with an additional qualifying term indicating the major defining feature of each separate type as it appears in the sequence noted above.

Diagnostic guidelines

None of the disorders in the group satisfies the criteria for either manic (F30.–) or depressive (F32.–) episodes, although emotional changes and individual affective symptoms may be prominent from time to time.

These disorders are also defined by the absence of organic causation, such as states of concussion, delirium, or dementia. Perplexity, preoccupation, and inattention to the immediate conversation are often present, but if they are so marked or persistent as to suggest delirium or dementia of organic cause, the diagnosis should be delayed until investigation or observation has clarified this point. Similarly, disorders in F23.– should not be diagnosed in the presence of obvious intoxication by drugs or alcohol. However, a recent minor increase in the consumption of, for instance, alcohol or marijuana, with no evidence of severe intoxication or disorientation, should not rule out the diagnosis of one of these acute psychotic disorders.

It is important to note that the 48-hour and the 2-week criteria are not put forward as the times of maximum severity and disturbance, but as times by which the psychotic symptoms have become obvious and disruptive of at least some aspects of daily life and work. The peak disturbance may be reached later in both instances; the symptoms and disturbance have only to be obvious by the stated times, in the sense that they will usually have brought the patient into contact with some form of helping or medical agency. Prodromal periods of anxiety, depression, social withdrawal, or mildly abnormal behaviour do not qualify for inclusion in these periods of time.

A fifth character may be used to indicate whether or not the acute psychotic disorder is associated with acute stress:

F23.x0 Without associated acute stress
F23.x1 With associated acute stress

F23.0 Acute polymorphic psychotic disorder without symptoms of schizophrenia

An acute psychotic disorder in which hallucinations, delusions, and perceptual disturbances are obvious but markedly variable, changing from day to day or even from hour to hour. Emotional turmoil, with intense transient feelings of happiness and ecstasy or anxieties and irritability, is also frequently present. This polymorphic and unstable, changing clinical picture is characteristic, and even though individual affective or psychotic symptoms may at times be present, the criteria for manic episode (F30.–), depressive episode (F32.–), or schizophrenia (F20.–) are not fulfilled. This disorder is particularly likely to have an abrupt onset (within 48 hours) and a rapid resolution of symptoms; in a large proportion of cases there is no obvious precipitating stress.

If the symptoms persist for more than 3 months, the diagnosis should be changed. (Persistent delusional disorder (F22.–) or other nonorganic psychotic disorder (F28) is likely to be the most appropriate.)

Diagnostic guidelines
For a definite diagnosis:

(a) the onset must be acute (from a nonpsychotic state to a clearly psychotic state within 2 weeks or less);
(b) there must be several types of hallucination or delusion, changing in both type and intensity from day to day or within the same day;
(c) there should be a similarly varying emotional state; and
(d) in spite of the variety of symptoms, none should be present with sufficient consistency to fulfil the criteria for schizophrenia (F20.–) or for manic or depressive episode (F30.– or F32.–).

Includes: bouffée délirante without symptoms of schizophrenia or unspecified
cycloid psychosis without symptoms of schizophrenia or unspecified

F23.1 Acute polymorphic psychotic disorder with symptoms of schizophrenia

An acute psychotic disorder which meets the descriptive criteria for acute polymorphic psychotic disorder (F23.0) but in which typically schizophrenic symptoms are also consistently present.

Diagnostic guidelines

For a definite diagnosis, criteria (a), (b), and (c) specified for acute polymorphic psychotic disorder (F23.0) must be fulfilled; in addition, symptoms that fulfil the criteria for schizophrenia (F20.–) must have been present for the majority of the time since the establishment of an obviously psychotic clinical picture.

If the schizophrenic symptoms persist for more than 1 month, the diagnosis should be changed to schizophrenia (F20.–).

Includes: bouffée délirante with symptoms of schizophrenia
cycloid psychosis with symptoms of schizophrenia

F23.2 Acute schizophrenia-like psychotic disorder

An acute psychotic disorder in which the psychotic symptoms are comparatively stable and fulfil the criteria for schizophrenia (F20.–) but have lasted for less than 1 month. Some degree of emotional variability or instability may be present, but not to the extent described in acute polymorphic psychotic disorder (F23.0).

Diagnostic guidelines

For a definite diagnosis:

(a) the onset of psychotic symptoms must be acute (2 weeks or less from a nonpsychotic to a clearly psychotic state);
(b) symptoms that fulfil the criteria for schizophrenia (F20.–) must have been present for the majority of the time since the establishment of an obviously psychotic clinical picture;
(c) the criteria for acute polymorphic psychotic disorder are not fulfilled.

If the schizophrenic symptoms last for more than 1 month, the diagnosis should be changed to schizophrenia (F20.–).

Includes: acute (undifferentiated) schizophrenia
brief schizophreniform disorder
brief schizophreniform psychosis
oneirophrenia
schizophrenic reaction

Excludes: organic delusional [schizophrenia-like] disorder (F06.2)
schizophreniform disorder NOS (F20.8)

F23.3 Other acute predominantly delusional psychotic disorders

Acute psychotic disorders in which comparatively stable delusions or hallucinations are the main clinical features, but do not fulfil the criteria for schizophrenia (F20.–). Delusions of persecution or reference are common, and hallucinations are usually auditory (voices talking directly to the patient).

Diagnostic guidelines

For a definite diagnosis:

(a) the onset of psychotic symptoms must be acute (2 weeks or less from a nonpsychotic to a clearly psychotic state);

(b) delusions or hallucinations must have been present for the majority of the time since the establishment of an obviously psychotic state; and

(c) the criteria for neither schizophrenia (F20.–) nor acute polymorphic psychotic disorder (F23.0) are fulfilled.

If delusions persist for more than 3 months, the diagnosis should be changed to persistent delusional disorder (F22.–). If only hallucinations persist for more than 3 months, the diagnosis should be changed to other nonorganic psychotic disorder (F28).

Includes: paranoid reaction
  psychogenic paranoid psychosis

F23.8 Other acute and transient psychotic disorders

Any other acute psychotic disorders that are unclassifiable under any other category in F23 (such as acute psychotic states in which definite delusions or hallucinations occur but persist for only small proportions of the time) should be coded here. States of undifferentiated excitement should also be coded here if more detailed information about the patient's mental state is not available, provided that there is no evidence of an organic cause.

F23.9 Acute and transient psychotic disorder, unspecified

Includes: (brief) reactive psychosis NOS

F24 Induced delusional disorder

A rare delusional disorder shared by two or occasionally more people with close emotional links. Only one person suffers from a genuine psychotic disorder; the delusions are induced in the other(s) and usually disappear when the people are separated. The psychotic illness of the dominant person is most commonly schizophrenic, but this is not necessarily or invariably so. Both the original delusions in the dominant person and the induced delusions are usually chronic and either persecutory or grandiose in nature. Delusional beliefs are transmitted this way only in uncommon circumstances. Almost invariably, the people concerned have an unusually close relationship and are isolated from others by language, culture, or geography. The individual in whom the delusions are induced is usually dependent on or subservient to the person with the genuine psychosis.

Diagnostic guidelines

A diagnosis of induced delusional disorder should be made only if:

(a) two or more people share the same delusion or delusional system and support one another in this belief;
(b) they have an unusually close relationship of the kind described above;
(c) there is temporal or other contextual evidence that the delusion was induced in the passive member(s) of the pair or group by contact with the active member.

Induced hallucinations are unusual but do not negate the diagnosis. However, if there are reasons for believing that two people living together have independent psychotic disorders neither should be coded here, even if some of the delusions are shared.

Includes: folie à deux
induced paranoid or psychotic disorder
symbiotic psychosis

Excludes: folie simultanée

F25 Schizoaffective disorders

These are episodic disorders in which both affective and schizophrenic symptoms are prominent within the same episode of illness, preferably simultaneously, but at least within a few days of each other. Their relationship to typical mood [affective] disorders (F30–F39) and to schizophrenic disorders (F20–F24) is uncertain. They are given a separate category because they are too common to be ignored. Other conditions in which affective symptoms are superimposed upon or form part of a pre-existing schizophrenic illness, or in which they coexist or alternate with other types of persistent delusional disorders, are classified under the appropriate category in F20–F29. Mood-incongruent delusions or hallucinations in affective disorders (F30.2, F31.2, F31.5, F32.3, or F33.3) do not by themselves justify a diagnosis of schizoaffective disorder.

Patients who suffer from recurrent schizoaffective episodes, particularly those whose symptoms are of the manic rather than the depressive type, usually make a full recovery and only rarely develop a defect state.

Diagnostic guidelines

A diagnosis of schizoaffective disorder should be made only when *both* definite schizophrenic and definite affective symptoms are prominent *simultaneously*, or within a few days of each other, within the same episode of illness, and when, as a consequence of this, the episode of illness does not meet criteria for either schizophrenia or a depressive or manic episode. The term should not be applied to patients who exhibit schizophrenic symptoms and affective symptoms only in different episodes of illness. It is common, for example, for a schizophrenic patient to present with depressive symptoms in the aftermath of a psychotic episode (see post-schizophrenic depression (F20.4)). Some patients have recurrent schizoaffective episodes, which may be of the manic or depressive type or a mixture of the two. Others have one or two schizoaffective episodes interspersed between typical episodes of mania or depression. In the former case, schizoaffective disorder is the appropriate diagnosis. In the latter, the occurrence of an occasional schizoaffective episode does not invalidate a diagnosis of bipolar affective disorder or recurrent depressive disorder if the clinical picture is typical in other respects.

F25.0 Schizoaffective disorder, manic type

A disorder in which schizophrenic and manic symptoms are both prominent in the same episode of illness. The abnormality of mood usually takes the form of elation, accompanied by increased self-esteem and grandiose ideas, but sometimes excitement or irritability are more obvious and accompanied by aggressive behaviour and persecutory ideas. In both cases there is increased energy, overactivity, impaired concentration, and a loss of normal social inhibition. Delusions of reference, grandeur, or persecution may be present, but other more typically schizophrenic symptoms are required to establish the diagnosis. People may insist, for example, that their thoughts are being broadcast or interfered with, or that alien forces are trying to control them, or they may report hearing voices of varied kinds or express bizarre delusional ideas that are not merely grandiose or persecutory. Careful questioning is often required to establish that an individual really is experiencing these morbid phenomena, and not merely joking or talking in metaphors. Schizoaffective disorders, manic type, are usually florid psychoses with an acute onset; although behaviour is often grossly disturbed, full recovery generally occurs within a few weeks.

Diagnostic guidelines

There must be a prominent elevation of mood, or a less obvious elevation of mood combined with increased irritability or excitement. Within the same episode, at least one and preferably two typically schizophrenic symptoms (as specified for schizophrenia (F20.–), diagnostic guidelines (a)–(d)) should be clearly present.

This category should be used both for a single schizoaffective episode of the manic type and for a recurrent disorder in which the majority of episodes are schizoaffective, manic type.

Includes: schizoaffective psychosis, manic type
schizophreniform psychosis, manic type

F25.1 Schizoaffective disorder, depressive type

A disorder in which schizophrenic and depressive symptoms are both prominent in the same episode of illness. Depression of mood is usually accompanied by several characteristic depressive symptoms or behavioural abnormalities such as retardation, insomnia, loss of energy, appetite or weight, reduction of normal interests, impairment of concentration, guilt, feelings of hopelessness, and suicidal thoughts. At the same time, or within the same episode, other more typically schizophrenic symptoms are present; patients may insist, for example, that their thoughts are being broadcast or interfered with, or that alien forces are trying to control them. They may be convinced that they are being spied upon or plotted against and this is not justified by their own behaviour. Voices may be heard that are not merely disparaging or condemnatory but that talk of killing the patient or discuss this behaviour between themselves. Schizoaffective episodes of the depressive type are usually less florid and alarming than schizoaffective episodes of the manic type, but they tend to last longer and the prognosis is less favourable. Although the majority of patients recover completely, some eventually develop a schizophrenic defect.

Diagnostic guidelines
There must be prominent depression, accompanied by at least two characteristic depressive symptoms or associated behavioural abnormalities as listed for depressive episode (F32.–); within the same episode, at least one and preferably two typically schizophrenic symptoms (as specified for schizophrenia (F20.–), diagnostic guidelines (a)–(d)) should be clearly present.

This category should be used both for a single schizoaffective episode, depressive type, and for a recurrent disorder in which the majority of episodes are schizoaffective, depressive type.

Includes: schizoaffective psychosis, depressive type
schizophreniform psychosis, depressive type

F25.2 Schizoaffective disorder, mixed type
Disorders in which symptoms of schizophrenia (F20.–) coexist with those of a mixed bipolar affective disorder (F31.6) should be coded here.

Includes: cyclic schizophrenia
mixed schizophrenic and affective psychosis

F25.8 Other schizoaffective disorders

F25.9 Schizoaffective disorder, unspecified

Includes: schizoaffective psychosis NOS

F28 Other nonorganic psychotic disorders

Psychotic disorders that do not meet the criteria for schizophrenia (F20.–) or for psychotic types of mood [affective] disorders (F30–F39), and psychotic disorders that do not meet the symptomatic criteria for persistent delusional disorder (F22.–) should be coded here.

Includes: chronic hallucinatory psychosis NOS

F29 Unspecified nonorganic psychosis

Includes: psychosis NOS
Excludes: mental disorder NOS (F99)
      organic or symptomatic psychosis NOS (F09)

Diagnostic criteria for research[1]

F20–F29 Schizophrenia, schizotypal and delusional disorders

F20 Schizophrenia

This overall category includes the common varieties of schizophrenia, together with some less common varieties and closely related disorders.

F20.0–F20.3 General criteria for paranoid, hebephrenic, catatonic, and undifferentiated schizophrenia

G1. Either *at least one* of the syndromes, symptoms, and signs listed under (1) below, *or* at least two of the symptoms and signs listed under (2) should be present for most of the time during an episode of psychotic illness lasting for at least 1 month (or at some time during most of the days).

(1) At least one of the following must be present:
   (a) thought echo, thought insertion or withdrawal, or thought broadcasting;
   (b) delusions of control, influence, or passivity, clearly referred to body or limb movements or specific thoughts, actions, or sensations; delusional perception;
   (c) hallucinatory voices giving a running commentary on the patient's behaviour, or discussing the patient among themselves, or other types of hallucinatory voices coming from some part of the body;
   (d) persistent delusions of other kinds that are culturally inappropriate and completely impossible (e.g. being able to control the weather, or being in communication with aliens from another world).

(2) *Or* at least two of the following:
   (a) persistent hallucinations in any modality, when occurring every day for at least 1 month, when accompanied by delusions (which may be fleeting or half-formed) without clear affective content, or when accompanied by persistent over-valued ideas;

---

[1]Reproduced from: *The ICD-10 Classification of Mental and Behavioural Disorders: diagnostic criteria for research*. Geneva, World Health Organization, 1993, pp. 64–76.

(b) neologisms, breaks, or interpolations in the train of thought, resulting in incoherence or irrelevant speech;

(c) catatonic behaviour, such as excitement, posturing or waxy flexibility, negativism, mutism, and stupor;

(d) "negative" symptoms, such as marked apathy, paucity of speech, and blunting or incongruity of emotional responses (it must be clear that these are not due to depression or to neuroleptic medication).

G2. *Most commonly used exclusion clauses*

(1) If the patient also meets criteria for manic episode (F30.–) or depressive episode (F32.–), the criteria listed under G1(1) and G1(2) above must have been met *before* the disturbance of mood developed.

(2) The disorder is not attributable to organic brain disease (in the sense of F00–F09), or to alcohol- or drug-related intoxication (F1x.0), dependence (F1x.2), or withdrawal (F1x.3 and F1x.4).

Comments   In evaluating the presence of these abnormal subjective experiences and behaviour, special care should be taken to avoid false-positive assessments, especially where culturally or subculturally influenced modes of expression and behaviour or a subnormal level of intelligence are involved.

Pattern of course

In view of the considerable variation of the course of schizophrenic disorders it may be desirable (especially for research) to specify the *pattern of course* by using a fifth character. Course should not usually be coded unless there has been a period of observation of at least 1 year.

F20.x0 Continuous
   No remission of psychotic symptoms throughout the period of observation.

F20.x1 Episodic with progressive deficit
   Progressive development of "negative" symptoms in the intervals between psychotic episodes.

F20.x2 Episodic with stable deficit
   Persistent but non-progressive "negative" symptoms in the intervals between psychotic episodes.

F20.x3 Episodic remittent
   Complete or virtually complete remissions between psychotic episodes.

F20.x4 Incomplete remission

F20.x5 Complete remission

F20.x8 Other

F20.x9 Course uncertain, period of observation too short

F20.0 Paranoid schizophrenia

A. The general criteria for schizophrenia (F20.0–F20.3) must be met.

B. Delusions or hallucinations must be prominent (such as delusions of persecution, reference, exalted birth, special mission, bodily change, or jealousy; threatening or commanding voices, hallucinations of smell or taste, sexual or other bodily sensations).

C. Flattening or incongruity of affect, catatonic symptoms, or incoherent speech must not dominate the clinical picture, although they may be present to a mild degree.

F20.1 Hebephrenic schizophrenia

A. The general criteria for schizophrenia (F20.0–F20.3) must be met.

B. Either of the following must be present:
  (1) definite and sustained flattening or shallowness of affect;
  (2) definite and sustained incongruity or inappropriateness of affect.

C. Either of the following must be present:
  (1) behaviour that is aimless and disjointed rather than goal-directed;
  (2) definite thought disorder, manifesting as speech that is disjointed, rambling, or incoherent.

D. Hallucinations or delusions must not dominate the clinical picture, although they may be present to a mild degree.

F20.2 Catatonic schizophrenia

A. The general criteria for schizophrenia (F20.0–F20.3) must eventually be met, although this may not be possible initially if the patient is uncommunicative.

B. For a period of at least 2 weeks one or more of the following catatonic behaviours must be prominent:
  (1) stupor (marked decrease in reactivity to the environment and reduction of spontaneous movements and activity) or mutism;
  (2) excitement (apparently purposeless motor activity, not influenced by external stimuli);
  (3) posturing (voluntary assumption and maintenance of inappropriate or bizarre postures);
  (4) negativism (an apparently motiveless resistance to all instructions or attempts to be moved, or movement in the opposite direction);
  (5) rigidity (maintenance of a rigid posture against efforts to be moved);
  (6) waxy flexibility (maintenance of limbs and body in externally imposed positions);
  (7) command automatism (automatic compliance with instructions).

F20.3 Undifferentiated schizophrenia

A. The general criteria for schizophrenia (F20.0–F20.3) must be met.

B. Either of the following must apply:
  (1) insufficient symptoms to meet the criteria for any of the subtypes F20.0, F20.1, F20.2, F20.4, or F20.5;

(2) so many symptoms that the criteria for more than one of the subtypes listed in (1) above are met.

F20.4 Post-schizophrenic depression

A. The general criteria for schizophrenia (F20.0–F20.3) must have been met within the past 12 months, but are not met at the present time.
B. One of the conditions in criterion G1(2) a, b, c, or d for F20.0–F20.3 must still be present.
C. The depressive symptoms must be sufficiently prolonged, severe, and extensive to meet criteria for at least a mild depressive episode (F32.0).

F20.5 Residual schizophrenia

A. The general criteria for schizophrenia (F20.0–F20.3) must have been met at some time in the past, but are not met at the present time.
B. At least four of the following "negative" symptoms have been present throughout the previous 12 months:
   (1) psychomotor slowing or underactivity;
   (2) definite blunting of affect;
   (3) passivity and lack of initiative;
   (4) poverty of either the quantity or the content of speech;
   (5) poor non-verbal communication by facial expression, eye contact, voice modulation, or posture;
   (6) poor social performance or self-care.

F20.6 Simple schizophrenia

A. There is slow but progressive development, over a period of at least 1 year, of all three of the following:
   (1) a significant and consistent change in the overall quality of some aspects of personal behaviour, manifest as loss of drive and interests, aimlessness, idleness, a self-absorbed attitude, and social withdrawal;
   (2) gradual appearance and deepening of "negative" symptoms such as marked apathy, paucity of speech, under-activity, blunting of affect, passivity and lack of initiative, and poor non-verbal communication (by facial expression, eye contact, voice modulation, and posture);
   (3) marked decline in social, scholastic, or occupational performance.
B. At no time are there any of the symptoms referred to in criterion G1 for F20.0–F20.3, nor are there hallucinations or well formed delusions of any kind, i.e. the individual must never have met the criteria for any other type of schizophrenia or for any other psychotic disorder.
C. There is no evidence of dementia or any other organic mental disorder listed in F00–F09.

F20.8 Other schizophrenia

F20.9 Schizophrenia, unspecified

F21 Schizotypal disorder

A. The subject must have manifested at least four of the following over a period of at least 2 years, either continuously or repeatedly:
   (1) inappropriate or constricted affect, with the individual appearing cold and aloof;
   (2) behaviour or appearance that is odd, eccentric, or peculiar;
   (3) poor rapport with others and a tendency to social withdrawal;
   (4) odd beliefs or magical thinking, influencing behaviour and inconsistent with subcultural norms;
   (5) suspiciousness or paranoid ideas;
   (6) ruminations without inner resistance, often with dysmorphophobic, sexual, or aggressive contents;
   (7) unusual perceptual experiences including somatosensory (bodily) or other illusions, depersonalization, or derealization;
   (8) vague, circumstantial, metaphorical, overelaborate, or often stereotyped thinking, manifested by odd speech or in other ways, without gross incoherence;
   (9) occasional transient quasi-psychotic episodes with intense illusions, auditory or other hallucinations, and delusion-like ideas, usually occurring without external provocation.
B. The subject must never have met the criteria for any disorder in F20.–(schizophrenia).

F22 Persistent delusional disorders

F22.0 Delusional disorder

A. A delusion or a set of related delusions, other than those listed as typically schizophrenic in criterion G1(1)b or d for F20.0–F20.3 (i.e. other than completely impossible or culturally inappropriate), must be present. The commonest examples are persecutory, grandiose, hypochondriacal, jealous (zelotypic), or erotic delusions.
B. The delusion(s) in criterion A must be present for at least 3 months.
C. The general criteria for schizophrenia (F20.0–F20.3) are not fulfilled.
D. There must be no persistent hallucinations in any modality (but there may be transitory or occasional auditory hallucinations that are not in the third person or giving a running commentary).
E. Depressive symptoms (or even a depressive episode (F32.–)) may be present intermittently, provided that the delusions persist at times when there is no disturbance of mood.
F. *Most commonly used exclusion clause.* There must be no evidence of primary or secondary organic mental disorder as listed under F00–F09, or of a psychotic disorder due to psychoactive substance use (F1x.5).

Specification for possible subtypes
The following types may be specified if desired: persecutory; litiginous; self-referential; grandiose; hypochondriacal (somatic); jealous; erotomanic.

F22.8 Other persistent delusional disorders
This is a residual category for persistent delusional disorders that do not meet the criteria for delusional disorder (F22.0). Disorders in which delusions are accompanied by persistent hallucinatory voices or by schizophrenic symptoms that are insufficient to meet criteria for schizophrenia (F20.–) should be coded here. Delusional disorders that have lasted for less than 3 months should, however, be coded, at least temporarily, under F23.–.

F22.9 Persistent delusional disorder, unspecified

F23 Acute and transient psychotic disorders

G1. There is acute onset of delusions, hallucinations, incomprehensible or incoherent speech, or any combination of these. The time interval between the first appearance of any psychotic symptoms and the presentation of the fully developed disorder should not exceed 2 weeks.

G2. If transient states of perplexity, misidentification, or impairment of attention and concentration are present, they do not fulfil the criteria for organically caused clouding of consciousness as specified for F05.–, criterion A.

G3. The disorder does not meet the symptomatic criteria for manic episode (F30.–), depressive episode (F32.–), or recurrent depressive disorder (F33.–).

G4. There is insufficient evidence of recent psychoactive substance use to fulfil the criteria for intoxication (F1x.0), harmful use (F1x.1), dependence (F1x.2), or withdrawal states (F1x.3 and F1x.4). The continued moderate and largely unchanged use of alcohol or drugs in amounts or with the frequency to which the individual is accustomed does not necessarily rule out the use of F23; this must be decided by clinical judgement and the requirements of the research project in question.

G5. *Most commonly used exclusion clause.* There must be no organic mental disorder (F00–F09) or serious metabolic disturbances affecting the central nervous system (this does not include childbirth).

A fifth character should be used to specify whether the acute onset of the disorder is associated with acute stress (occurring 2 weeks or less before evidence of first psychotic symptoms):

F23.x0 Without associated acute stress
F23.x1 With associated acute stress

For research purposes it is recommended that change of the disorder from a non-psychotic to a clearly psychotic state is further specified as either abrupt (onset within 48 hours) or acute (onset in more than 48 hours but less than 2 weeks).

F23.0 Acute polymorphic psychotic disorder without symptoms of schizophrenia

A. The general criteria for acute and transient psychotic disorders (F23) must be met.
B. Symptoms change rapidly in both type and intensity from day to day or within the same day.
C. Any type of either hallucinations or delusions occurs, for at least several hours, at any time from the onset of the disorder.
D. Symptoms from at least two of the following categories occur at the same time:
    (1) emotional turmoil, characterized by intense feelings of happiness or ecstasy, or overwhelming anxiety or marked irritability;
    (2) perplexity, or misidentification of people or places;
    (3) increased or decreased motility, to a marked degree.
E. If any of the symptoms listed for schizophrenia (F20.0–F20.3), criterion $G(1)$ and (2), are present, they are present only for a minority of the time from the onset, i.e. criterion B of F23.1 is not fulfilled.
F. The total duration of the disorder does not exceed 3 months.

F23.1 Acute polymorphic psychotic disorder with symptoms of schizophrenia

A. Criteria A, B, C, and D of acute polymorphic psychotic disorder (F23.0) must be met.
B. Some of the symptoms for schizophrenia (F20.0–F20.3) must have been present for the majority of the time since the onset of the disorder, although the full criteria need not be met, i.e. at least one of the symptoms in criteria $G1(1)a$ to $G1(2)c$.
C. The symptoms of schizophrenia in criterion B above do not persist for more than 1 month.

F23.2 Acute schizophrenia-like psychotic disorder

A. The general criteria for acute and transient psychotic disorders (F23) must be met.
B. The criteria for schizophrenia (F20.0–F20.3) are met, with the exception of the criterion for duration.
C. The disorder does not meet criteria B, C, and D for acute polymorphic psychotic disorder (F23.0).
D. The total duration of the disorder does not exceed 1 month.

F23.3 Other acute predominantly delusional psychotic disorders

A. The general criteria for acute and transient psychotic disorders (F23) must be met.

B. Relatively stable delusions and/or hallucinations are present but do not fulfil the symptomatic criteria for schizophrenia (F20.0–F20.3).
C. The disorder does not meet the criteria for acute polymorphic psychotic disorder (F23.0).
D. The total duration of the disorder does not exceed 3 months.

F23.8 Other acute and transient psychotic disorders

Any other acute psychotic disorders that are not classifiable under any other category in F23 (such as acute psychotic states in which definite delusions or hallucinations occur but persist for only small proportions of the time) should be coded here. States of undifferentiated excitement should also be coded here if more detailed information about the patient's mental state is not available, provided that there is no evidence of an organic cause.

F23.9 Acute and transient psychotic disorder, unspecified

F24 Induced delusional disorder

A. The individual(s) must develop a delusion or delusional system originally held by someone else with a disorder classified in F20–F23.
B. The people concerned must have an unusually close relationship with one another, and be relatively isolated from other people.
C. The individual(s) must not have held the belief in question before contact with the other person, and must not have suffered from any other disorder classified in F20–F23 in the past.

F25 Schizoaffective disorders

Note. This diagnosis depends upon an approximate "balance" between the number, severity, and duration of the schizophrenic and affective symptoms.

G1. The disorder meets the criteria for one of the affective disorders (F30.–, F31.–, F32.–) of moderate or severe degree, as specified for each category.
G2. Symptoms from at least one of the groups listed below must be clearly present for most of the time during a period of at least 2 weeks (these groups are almost the same as for schizophrenia (F20.0–F20.3)):

(1) thought echo, thought insertion or withdrawal, thought broadcasting (criterion G1(1)a for F20.0–F20.3);
(2) delusions of control, influence, or passivity, clearly referred to body or limb movements or specific thoughts, actions, or sensations (criterion G1(1)b for F20.0–F20.3);
(3) hallucinatory voices giving a running commentary on the patient's behaviour or discussing the patient among themselves, or other types of hallucinatory voices coming from some part of the body (criterion G1(1)c for F20.0–F20.3);

(4) persistent delusions of other kinds that are culturally inappropriate and completely impossible, but not merely grandiose or persecutory (criterion G1(1)d for F20.0–F20.3), e.g. has visited other worlds; can control the clouds by breathing in and out; can communicate with plants or animals without speaking;

(5) grossly irrelevant or incoherent speech, or frequent use of neologisms (a marked form of criterion G1(2)b for F20.0–F20.3);

(6) intermittent but frequent appearance of some forms of catatonic behaviour, such as posturing, waxy flexibility, and negativism (criterion G1(2)c for F20.0–F20.3).

G3. Criteria G1 and G2 above must be met within the same episode of the disorder, and concurrently for at least part of the episode. Symptoms from both G1 and G2 must be prominent in the clinical picture.

G4. *Most commonly used exclusion clause.* The disorder is not attributable to organic mental disorder (in the sense of F00–F09), or to psychoactive substance-related intoxication, dependence, or withdrawal (F10–F19).

F25.0 Schizoaffective disorder, manic type

A. The general criteria for schizoaffective disorder (F25) must be met.

B. Criteria for a manic disorder (F30.1 or F31.1) must be met.

F25.1 Schizoaffective disorder, depressive type

A. The general criteria for schizoaffective disorder (F25) must be met.

B. The criteria for a depressive disorder of at least moderate severity (F31.3, F31.4, F32.1 or F32.2) must be met.

F25.2 Schizoaffective disorder, mixed type

A. The general criteria for schizoaffective disorder (F25) must be met.

B. The criteria for mixed bipolar affective disorder (F31.6) must be met.

F25.8 Other schizoaffective disorders

F25.9 Schizoaffective disorder, unspecified

Comments If desired, further subtypes of schizoaffective disorder may be specified, according to the longitudinal development of the disorder, as follows:

F25.x0 Concurrent affective and schizophrenic symptoms only Symptoms as defined in criterion G2 for F25.

F25.x1 Concurrent affective and schizophrenic symptoms, plus persistence of schizophrenic symptoms beyond the duration of affective symptoms

F28 Other nonorganic psychotic disorders

Psychotic disorders that do not meet the criteria for schizophrenia (F20.0–F20.3) or for psychotic types of mood [affective] disorders (F30–F39), and psychotic disorders that do not meet the symptomatic criteria for persistent delusional disorder (F22.–) should be coded here (persistent hallucinatory disorder is an example). Combinations of symptoms not covered by the previous categories F20–F25, such as delusions other than those listed as typically schizophrenic under criterion G1(1)b or d for F20.0–F20.3 (i.e. other than completely impossible or culturally inappropriate) plus catatonia, should also be included here.

F29 Unspecified nonorganic psychosis

7